REGULAR

REGULAR

*The Ultimate Guide to Taming
Unruly Bowels and Achieving Inner Peace*

Tamara Duker Freuman
MS, RD, CDN

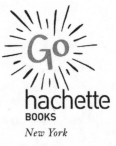

hachette
BOOKS
New York

Hachette Go, an imprint of Hachette Books
Hachette Book Group
1290 Avenue of the Americas
New York, NY 10104
HachetteGo.com
Facebook.com/HachetteGo
Instagram.com/HachetteGo

First Edition: April 2023

Hachette Books is a division of Hachette Book Group, Inc.

The Hachette Go and Hachette Books name and logos are trademarks of Hachette Book Group, Inc.

The Hachette Speakers Bureau provides a wide range of authors for speaking events.

To find out more, go to www.hachettespeakersbureau.com or call (866) 376-6591.

Hachette Go books may be purchased in bulk for business, educational, or promotional use. For information, please contact your local bookseller or Hachette Book Group Special Markets Department at: special.markets@hbgusa.com.

The publisher is not responsible for websites (or their content) that are not owned by the publisher.

Print book interior design by Jeff Williams

Library of Congress Cataloging-in-Publication Data

Name: Freuman, Tamara Duker, author.
Title: Regular: the ultimate guide to taming unruly bowels and achieving inner peace / Tamara Duker Freuman, MS, RD, CDN.
Description: New York: Hachette Go, [2023] | Includes bibliographical references and index.
Identifiers: LCCN 2022037815 | ISBN 9780306830785 (hardcover) | ISBN 9780306830792 (paperback) | ISBN 9780306830808 (ebook)
Subjects: LCSH: Gastrointestinal system—Diseases—Popular works. | Gastrointestinal system—Diseases—Prevention—Popular works. | Gastrointestinal system—Diseases—Diet therapy—Popular works.
Classification: LCC RC806 .F74 2023 | DDC 616.3/3—dc23/eng/20221202

LC record available at https://lccn.loc.gov/2022037815

ISBNs: 978-0-306-83078-5 (hardcover); 978-0-306-83080-8 (ebook)

Printed in the United States of America

LSC-C

Printing 1, 2023

To Eric and Yevgenia, the two best work spouses I could ever ask for, with gratitude for all that you have taught me, for your friendship, and for the phenomenal potty humor along the way

The abdomen is the reason why man does not easily take himself for a god.

—FRIEDRICH NIETZSCHE, *Beyond Good and Evil*

Contents

PART I

Introduction

poo•pho•ria \pü-fō-rē-ə\ noun
a feeling of elation and inner peace
following completion of an easy-to-pass
and fully relieving bowel movement

What's Normal?

Defining Regularity and Irregularity

IT GOES BY MANY NAMES. In polite company, it's referred to as stool, feces, or a **bowel movement**—and in truly polite company, it's not referred to at all. Among friends and family, we may call it by nicknames like doody, poo, poop, or number two. Or we may allude to its taking place using one of hundreds of euphemisms like "seeing a man about a horse" or "laying a brick." Just as the Inuit have dozens of names for snow as a sign of its centrality to their way of life, humans in many societies have dozens of words to refer to the waste that we pass from our digestive systems—and the act of doing it. Whether or not we care to admit it, moving our bowels is a pretty central and universal aspect of our human experience—and this is particularly evident when our bowels aren't behaving themselves.

What Is Stool?

It seems fitting to start off a book about digestive **regularity** with some basic definitions: What, exactly, is this stuff coming out of our anuses? Stool—or poop, or whatever your preferred term—is a waste product that comes together in the penultimate portion of our digestive tract called the **colon**—or large intestine. It's composed of a variety of ingredients, including:

Water

About 75% of your **stool** is composed of water, with the remainder composed of various solid matter as described below. The longer a stool spends in your colon, the less water it will contain. This is because as the waste stream makes its way through the colon, some fluid and sodium are reabsorbed back into the body. It explains why people with slower "transit times" will have harder stools, and why people with faster transit times have looser, more watery stools.

Leftover Residue from Your Diet

Any portions of your food that were unable to be broken down (digested) and absorbed into the body farther upstream in the small intestine will proceed onward to the colon for elimination. Mostly, this includes indigestible plant fibers: corn kernels and the skins of tomatoes, peas, and peppers; wheat bran; spinach leaves and chewed- up romaine hearts; fruit skins from blueberries, grapes, and apples; flax, poppy, and kiwi seeds; popcorn kernel hulls and poorly chewed nut pieces. The list goes on. Basically, any plant-based fiber that we humans don't have enzymes to digest will fulfill its destiny as residue that bulks up our stool. It is perfectly normal—and indeed, expected—to see these fibers in your stool.

Dead Bacteria

A sizable percentage of the solid part of your stool is composed of dead bacteria. Our digestive tract is home to trillions of microorganisms that are collectively known as the **gut microbiota**—and the vast majority of them are concentrated in the colon. Bacterial populations are constantly in flux—with older organisms dying off to be replaced by newly divided ones. The dead ones enter our waste stream and get pooped out. Because dead bacteria still contain their genetic material, scientists using specific types of gene tests on stool samples can actually identify some of the characteristics of each person's unique gut microbiota—garnering information on a subset of the species and strains that actually live in our colons and in what relative proportions. The composition of a person's gut microbiota is as individual as their fingerprints.

Pigments from Dead Red Blood Cells

We have trillions of red blood cells, and when they die, our body needs to discard their little corpses so they don't pile up. Waste products from these dead cells travel to the liver and become transformed into a pigment called bilirubin, which is packaged up into a digestive fluid called bile and released into the intestines as part of the digestive process. Some of the bilirubin pigment from bile remains in the digestive tract and travels on to the colon, where it's acted upon by the resident gut bacteria; this turns their yellowish color to a darker brown color and gives stool its signature brownish hue. When stool rushes through the colon rapidly, before the bacteria have an opportunity to work their magic on these pigments, you may wind up with lighter colored stools—yellowy or orangey or lighter brown.

Other Stuff

The cells lining the colon secrete small amounts of other stuff into stool, including some proteins and mucus; when these cells themselves die and are shed, they become one with the poop as well. There's a wee bit of fat in the stool as well—but there shouldn't be all that much. Excessively fatty stools are typically a sign of malabsorption, which is discussed further in Chapter 6. Finally, there are minute amounts of minerals and **electrolytes**, such as calcium, sodium, phosphate, iron, potassium, magnesium, and zinc.

What Does It Mean to Be "Regular"?

In the gastroenterology practice where I work, patients often want to know how their pooping patterns stack up against those of other people. Really what they're asking is: "Am I normal?" It's a difficult question to answer because there is a range of elimination habits that would be considered normal—and the quantitative stats (number of poops per day or week) don't always convey the qualitative information (ease of passing poops, how you feel before and after pooping episodes) that is necessary to determine whether your experience is, indeed, normal.

CONSTIPATION

- Fewer than three spontaneous bowel movements per week

- Straining to pass stool at least 25% of the time

- Hard lumpy stools (type 1 or type 2 on Bristol Stool Chart; see below)

- Feeling incompletely emptied out at least 25% of the time

- Needing to resort to manual maneuvers to help move your bowels

Source: Rome IV Criteria

In terms of frequency, the range of what's considered normal can roughly be summed up as anything from four bowel movements per day to three bowel movements per week. Having more than four bowel movements daily is sometimes referred to as **hyperdefecation**, whereas going less than three times per week would meet one of the clinical definitions of **constipation**. Very frequent—but formed—stools are not actually necessarily considered diarrhea. **Diarrhea** has as much to do with frequency or volume as it does with texture. By the book, diarrhea is defined as loose, watery stools at least three times per day, or stool volume in excess of 250 mL per day (as if any of us measure it!). In reality, though, if you were having watery stools "only" twice per day, it's still going to be considered diarrhea clinically.

But before you start panicking as you compare your pooping frequency with the range described above, ask yourself one additional, important question: **Does your pooping frequency pose a problem for you?** For example, you may follow an incredibly high-fiber diet that causes you to poop four or more times daily, but your stools are perfectly formed, easy to pass, not urgent, and unaccompanied by problematic symptoms. On the flip side, you may only go twice per week—but you don't experience any discomfort in between pooping episodes, and each time you go, you pass a significant amount of stool in long, easy-to-pass bowel movements that leave you with a terrific sense of relief. In terms of frequency, both of these scenarios fall out of the range of what's considered normal, but that doesn't mean that they require an intervention to modify the frequency of things. As my gastroenterologist colleague is fond of saying, your pooping "is only a problem for you if it's a problem for you." Or, if it ain't broke, don't fix it.

Now, compare these scenarios with someone whose pooping frequency may fall within the normal range, but who's perfectly miserable nonetheless. Perhaps you experience pain, cramping, or bloating associated with defecating. Or maybe you go two to three times daily, but each time you go, only tiny, hard little balls come out—denying you any sense of relief. Which scenario would be preferable: the "abnormally" frequent/infrequent pooper who feels perfectly fine, or the person who poops with "normal" frequency but suffers feelings of bloating, discomfort, pain, or incomplete relief? Clearly, measuring frequency of pooping doesn't tell the whole story, and tweaking your diet or bowel regimen just to hack the frequency of your bowel movements for frequency's sake alone probably isn't necessary.

The Bristol Stool Chart

The quality, quantity, and frequency of your stools are considered in establishing whether you have constipation or diarrhea.

To evaluate stool quality and help you convey what's happening in the bathroom, some clinicians refer to the **Bristol Stool Chart**— so named for the Bristol Royal Infirmary in England that was home to the clinician who developed it in the late 1990s, Dr. Ken Heaton. The Bristol Stool Chart is an illustrated scale of bowel movements that represent the full range of human output: from highly constipated, hard little balls (what I often refer to as rabbit pellets) to liquidy, watery diarrhea . . . and the various possibilities in between. It first appeared in Dr. Heaton's book, *Understanding Your Bowels*, published in 1999 in the United Kingdom by Family Doctor Publications.

The first instinct many of my patients have when seeing the Bristol chart for the first time is to worry that their stools don't always (or ever) look like type 3 or type 4. So it needs to be said that the Bristol scale is not intended to offer up a paradigm to which we are all supposed to aspire. Rather, it is a descriptive tool initially intended for research purposes, and now best used to help patients convey what their output looks like so that a doctor can make some educated guesses about what may be going on inside. This is especially important because patients routinely use the words *diarrhea* and *constipation* in subjective ways that do not necessarily correlate with stool form. Often, my patients will tell me they have "diarrhea," but what they actually mean is that they have too-frequent and too-urgent bowel movements, even though the stools themselves are relatively formed (say, like type 5 on the Bristol scale). Similarly, I've had patients tell me they are constipated, but their stools are actually quite soft. What they're actually describing is a situation in which they have to strain even to push out these soft stools, or a feeling like they are not able to "get everything out." By using the Bristol Stool Chart as a descriptive tool instead of more subjectively applied terms like "diarrhea" and "constipation," clinicians can better understand what might be happening inside the body and zero in on the right solution more quickly.

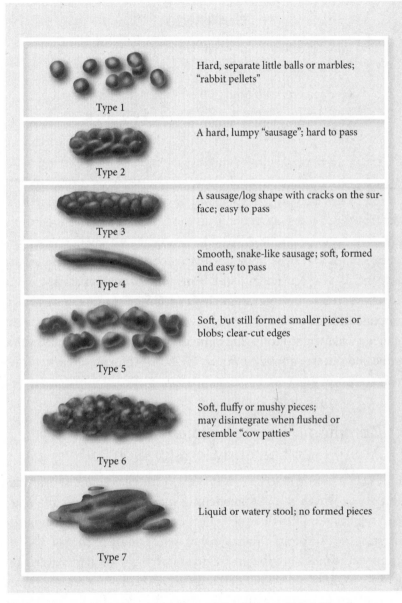

Type 1 — Hard, separate little balls or marbles; "rabbit pellets"

Type 2 — A hard, lumpy "sausage"; hard to pass

Type 3 — A sausage/log shape with cracks on the surface; easy to pass

Type 4 — Smooth, snake-like sausage; soft, formed and easy to pass

Type 5 — Soft, but still formed smaller pieces or blobs; clear-cut edges

Type 6 — Soft, fluffy or mushy pieces; may disintegrate when flushed or resemble "cow patties"

Type 7 — Liquid or watery stool; no formed pieces

FIGURE 1-1: Artist's Reproduction of the Bristol Stool Chart

Artwork by Mehtonen Medical Studios

DIARRHEA

- Loose, watery stools (type 6 or type 7 on the Bristol Stool Chart) that occur three or more times per day

- Or passing more than 200 g of stool per day (about 7 oz.)—though most people don't weigh their stools to track this!

All of this is to say that the goal is *not* for everyone's poop to look like type 3 or type 4 on the scale all the time. There is no such thing as a perfect poop, and healthy poops come in a variety of colors, textures, shapes, and sizes. Your stools are not contestants in any beauty pageant. If you are feeling well and your bathroom habits aren't causing you any trouble, then there's no need to tinker with diet, supplements, or medications just to change the appearance of your bowel movements. However, chances are if you've purchased this book, then there's probably room for improvement when it comes to your bowel function.

Common Misconceptions About Diarrhea and Constipation

The fact of having diarrhea gives only a limited amount of information about what's actually happening inside the body. While diarrhea typically implies that the transit time of your poop through the intestines is more rapid than normal, you cannot draw conclusions about where in the gut the problem underlying your diarrhea is originating. In most cases—but certainly not all—the root cause of diarrhea is in the colon, which is the large intestine. By the time your gut's contents have arrived to the colon, virtually all the absorbable nutrients have long since been taken up in the small intestine: calories from carbs, proteins, and fats; vitamins; and minerals. The leftover stuff—all that fibrous residue described earlier—is deposited

into the waste stream on a journey through the colon to be eliminated. As the waste stream makes its way through the colon, some
fluid and sodium are reabsorbed back into the body. This results in
the mushy waste turning firmer, into more formed stool.

When waste is rushed through the colon faster than usual—
as may be the case for many types of diarrhea discussed in this
book—there's not enough time for all the fluid (and electrolytes like
sodium) to be reabsorbed. In other cases, inflammation in the colon
can cause the cells lining it to secrete excess water and electrolytes
into the **bowel**, which similarly results in diarrhea. Both cases result
in the loose—sometimes even watery—character of diarrhea. (If the
transit time through the colon is too rushed to enable the pigments
to undergo bacterial transformation, the stool may be a lighter color
than usual as well—more of an orangey color than a true brown.)
However, other than fluid and sodium, this type of diarrhea involves
little to no nutrient malabsorption. As you will learn in Chapter 2,
your carbs, fats, proteins, vitamins, and minerals have long since
been absorbed in the small intestine before arriving to the colon!
When diarrhea originates in the colon, therefore, there should be
minimal to no weight loss—unless, of course, your fear of having
diarrhea or just generally feeling digestively unsettled leads you to
eat less than usual, which is certainly often the case.

I make this point for a few reasons. One, because there's a common misconception among my patients with **chronic diarrhea**
that their bodies are not absorbing any nutrients ("Everything goes
right through me"). **As a very general rule, if you're having diarrhea regularly but are not losing weight, then you're probably
absorbing your nutrients (except possibly some electrolytes)
just fine.** There are certainly some exceptions to this rule, particularly if you have Crohn's disease (Chapter 7) or celiac disease (Chapter 6). But the majority of causes of diarrhea taken up in this book
do not result in meaningful malabsorption of vitamins or minerals
when there is not accompanying weight loss.

Two, many people believe that if they see fiber in their diarrheal
stools—veggie skins, nut particles, seeds, and the like—that this is a

sign they have an intolerance to them, or that they are not absorbing the nutrients in these foods. This is also untrue. **No one can digest fiber.** That's what makes it fiber. Anyone who eats corn or tomatoes or blueberries *will* have the skins wind up in their stool. But when waste takes its time moving through the colon, these fibrous particles are less visible to us because (a) their colors are muted by the transformative effect of bacterial action, and (b) they're often buried deep inside a formed log of stool. In contrast, a loose stool means that dietary fiber will be more visible in the toilet as bits of waste break apart and put them on display.

On to the next misconception about **irregularity**: the conflation of digestion and metabolism. Diarrhea and constipation both result from factors that affect the transit time of food and waste through your intestines, many of which will be explored in great detail throughout the rest of this book. Often, however, I encounter patients who believe that their bowel function is a proxy for their metabolism—having diarrhea, for example, means that one has a "fast metabolism" while constipation suggests one has a "slow metabolism." This is not accurate. I suspect one of the things fueling this misconception is the phenomenon of seeing certain recognizable dietary components in your poop mere hours after eating it. *If that corn I ate at lunch is already in my poop at bedtime*, you think to yourself, *that must mean I burned all that corn's calories up lickety-split*! Perhaps, then, it's worth taking a moment to explain the differences between digestive system transit time and metabolism—and why they're not synonymous.

Your rate of **digestion** is measured in units of time: how long it takes food to travel from your mouth, down through the esophagus (food pipe), into the stomach, through each of the three segments of your small intestine—and then for the residual waste to continue traveling through the colon and out your anus into the toilet bowl. (The sum total of this journey is called oroanal transit time in clinical circles.) The term "metabolism" describes the process by which the cells of our body convert the food we eat into usable energy, and it is measured in terms of calories (energy) expended. Metabolism does not take place in the digestive tract, but rather inside each and every cell of the body as nutrients absorbed from the digestive tract are delivered to them by the bloodstream and converted into usable energy. Your metabolism can be thought of as how your cells utilize the energy you've absorbed from the digestive tract.

Metabolism is typically talked about in terms of the "metabolic rate," which is how many calories you need to maintain your current body's many functions without gaining or losing any weight *while you are at rest*. When people refer to a "fast metabolism," it's usually code for they burn through lots of calories to maintain their weight. When they refer to a "slow metabolism," it typically refers to the opposite—they maintain their weight at relatively fewer calories.

The rate of your digestion is not necessarily related to the rate of your metabolism. For example, waste may move through your colon quickly, making you prone to diarrhea due to a rapid intestinal transit time, while your body's cells are relatively efficient with their energy use, meaning you also maintain your weight at a low calorie intake—or have what's considered a slow metabolism. The opposite scenario can also be true: you can be constipated due to a slow intestinal transit time, but still enjoy the ability to eat a lot of calories and not gain weight due to a fast metabolism.

However, I say that the rate of digestion is not necessarily related to the rate of your metabolism because, in some cases, dysfunction of your thyroid can cause slowdowns or speedups of *both* your digestion and your metabolism, in which case the two processes are correlated. But apart from the case of underactive or overactive thyroid function, there's not a whole lot of overlap between factors that influence the rate of your digestion and metabolism, respectively. These are completely separate bodily processes, with your metabolic rate governed by things like age, sex, height, weight, body composition (amount of muscle mass), levels of many different hormone levels—and even body temperature. The rate of your digestive transit can be influenced by certain and sometimes overlapping hormone levels, but also things like the textural and nutritional composition of your meal; dedicated pacemaker cells in the stomach; the function of various nerves that communicate with the smooth muscles lining the digestive tract; and the length of your intestines, among others. Digestive transit is discussed in more detail in the next chapter.

When it comes to misconceptions about constipation in particular (shall we call them "mis-consticeptions"?), one that I hear often is a fear that constipation is dangerous because "when food sits around too long in the gut, it rots [putrefies] and releases toxins." There's so much that is wrong with this statement. For starters, since constipation happens in the colon, there is no food arriving there. Any food that was digestible has long since been broken down enzymatically in your small intestine, its building blocks absorbed from the gut into the bloodstream for distribution throughout the body. Foods like intact meat or whole fruit that we think of as being able to "rot" (a nonscientific term that refers to decay by microorganisms) are not actually making it all the way to your colon. Whatever makes it to the colon is indigestible residue from the foods we eat—mostly fiber—which is waste on arrival. While it is true—and beneficial— that the fiber in our waste is acted upon by bacteria in our colon, the correct way to describe this process is "fermentation"—not "rotting" or "putrefaction."

Fermentation is what happens when bacteria degrade carbohydrates like the fibers, starches, and indigestible sugars that resist digestion and absorption in the small intestine. And when certain bacteria engage in fermentation of carbohydrates like fiber in our guts, they release very beneficial compounds called short-chain fatty acids (SCFAs)—not detrimental toxins. In other words, fermentation of our high-fiber waste is generally the sign of something health-promoting going on. The microscopic inhabitants of our colons will also produce various gases, including hydrogen and sometimes methane. These gases are not inherently bad or toxic—no matter what their smell might lead you to believe—though having higher levels of methane gas in the colon does seem to be associated with constipation. If you ever come across anyone using the terms "rotting" and "putrefaction" to describe anything related to digestion, it should serve as a red flag that there's some nonscientific fearmongering going on. In fact, the colon has evolved to handle all these by-products of bacterial activity, and they are only toxic if they escape into your bloodstream.

Why Is It Important to Remedy Diarrhea or Constipation?

While the discussion on misconceptions above is meant to put your mind at ease about some of the more unfounded fears about diarrhea and constipation, I don't mean to imply that there are no health risks associated with chronic diarrhea or chronic constipation. There certainly can be. Getting regular is a worthwhile health goal so as to minimize the risk of a variety of common irregularity-related conditions, including some of the more common ones discussed in this chapter.

Hemorrhoids

Hemorrhoids are cushions filled with veins in your anal canal; when they become swollen, they can cause uncomfortable symptoms and even bleeding. Symptomatic hemorrhoids are generally associated with chronic constipation, as the constant straining to pass stool can put excess pressure on the delicate blood vessels down there and cause them to bulge. However, it's not unheard of for people with hyperdefecation—or excessively frequent bowel movements—to develop symptomatic hemorrhoids, too. Frequent trips to the bathroom and lots of sitting on the toilet can create the kind of wear and tear that predisposes to symptomatic hemorrhoids. In fact, anything that places excess pressure on these blood vessels can cause swelling. Pregnancy commonly results in symptomatic hemorrhoids—both from the excess weight placing significant downward pressure on your nether region and from the pushing during delivery itself. Habitual, prolonged sitting on the toilet that's unproductive can also result in symptomatic hemorrhoids—say, while answering e-mails, playing Wordle on your phone, or doing a crossword puzzle. In fact,

anything that results in forceful bearing down can result in a bulging hemorrhoid. When I was in my twenties and well before I had
my children, I actually developed one in an attempt to do a pull-up
at the gym! (No good deed goes unpunished, apparently.)

Hemorrhoids come in two varieties: internal and external. When
they're internal, you won't see them, but they may make their presence known in other ways. If you're lucky, they'll often just leave the
occasional spot of blood on your toilet paper after wiping. For some
people, they can cause significant pain, pressure, or even obstructive
symptoms. In serious cases, internal hemorrhoids may cause enough
bleeding so as to result in anemia-provoking iron losses—and this
can be especially so for people who use blood-thinning medications
that make it difficult to stop bleeding. External hemorrhoids are
generally more noticeable; they can look like little bulging bubbles
or mini clusters of grapes dangling out of your anus. Sometimes
they itch or hurt, and often they make wiping yourself clean after a
bowel movement a very tricky thing to do. If external hemorrhoids
become acutely thrombosed—filled with a blood clot—they can
also bleed. These symptoms can be mild to severe. In severe cases, it
can hurt to even sit. (A donut chair cushion helps.)

Hemorrhoids can be treated with topical medications to help
shrink them and alleviate the pain and itchiness, to varying degrees of
effectiveness—both prescription and over-the-counter options are
available. Preparation H (phenylephrine HCl) is a common brand
marketed here in the United States whose active ingredient helps to
shrink blood vessels while its inactive ingredients coat and protect
the delicate skin. Wet wipes soaked in witch hazel can help you get
clean after a bowel movement without excessive dry wiping that can
aggravate hemorrhoids even further; this is essentially what Tucks
Medicated Cooling Pads and their generic store-brand equivalents
are. Many people with chronic symptomatic hemorrhoids find that
investing in a bidet attachment for their toilet is very worthwhile;
this device directs a stream of water to your backside while sitting on
the toilet to help gently clean you after having a bowel movement
and avoid the need for more abrasive dry wiping. **Sitz baths** are

little plastic bedpan-looking things that you can attach to your toilet seat so as to give your bottom a brief, pain-relieving soak without having to fill the entire bathtub. More problematic cases of internal hemorrhoids are often handled with medical procedures like banding, in which a doctor essentially ties a rubber band around the base of the hemorrhoid to cut off its blood supply until it shrivels up. When banding fails or can't be done, a surgery called hemorrhoidectomy can be done under anesthesia to cut off the hemorrhoid. It can be quite a painful recovery.

If all this sounds miserable and best avoided if possible, then consider hemorrhoid risk reduction as one great motivator to get regular—and stay that way.

Diverticular Disease

Diverticular disease is what happens when your colon develops little bulges in its inner lining that protrude outward toward the muscle layer. These are called **diverticula**—and they're basically pocket-like hernias where stool can get trapped as it moves through. Having these pouches is called **diverticulosis**—and it's typically asymptomatic. But up to a quarter of people with diverticulosis will develop a complication called **diverticulitis**, an infection of their diverticula. Mild cases of diverticulitis involve fever, acute pain, and a change in bowel habits; it's typically treated with bowel rest (no solid food) for a few days, possibly followed by antibiotics to treat the infection if your liquid diet doesn't quiet things down. Severe or recurrent cases may require surgery to cut out the affected section of the colon to prevent complications like excessive bleeding, bowel perforations, or abscesses. If even a mild case of diverticulitis doesn't sound like your cup of tea, then it's all the more reason to work on getting more regular in the bathroom.

While researchers aren't entirely clear about how diverticula develop, they're thought to result from increased pressure within the colon—such as from chronic straining to move your bowels or from a diet low in fiber that therefore requires the colon to exert more force to propel waste forward. Western-style toilets are a known risk factor for developing diverticula; there is significantly less diverticular disease in societies where squat toilets (or just squatting to poop) are the standard. There may be other factors at play—such as weakened connective tissue that makes these herniations more likely to occur. Having irritable bowel syndrome (IBS; Chapter 4), chronic constipation, and a low-fiber diet are all risk factors for diverticular disease, as are the following: smoking, having a higher body mass index, lack of exercise, and overuse of nonsteroidal anti-inflammatory drugs (NSAIDs) or opioid painkillers.

Anal Fissures

An **anal fissure** is a small tear in the skin lining your anus. But just as a teensy little paper cut can be disproportionately painful, so, too, can a small anal fissure wreak havoc on your life. For starters, the moist tissue that lines your anus is full of nerves, so fissures can be extremely painful, especially as bowel movements rub up against them on the way out, and the pain can persist for hours after completing a bowel movement. Secondly, since fissures are essentially little cuts located on the moist skin that lines a muscle that expands often and is situated smack in the middle of your body's waste stream, they can take a while to heal—sometimes weeks . . . or months . . . or never.

Hard stools that require lots of straining to pass are more likely to contribute to an anal fissure, though some people with chronic diarrhea can develop one as well as the result of excessive wear and tear on the delicate anal tissue. Once you have a fissure, you'll need to engage in a delicate dance of eating enough fiber to soften your bowel movements and minimize straining, but not so much that you're going to the bathroom so often that it aggravates the fissure further. You'll likely rely on prescription topical medications and/or sitz baths (see above) for pain relief—and in some cases, even oral medications are required to reduce anal spasms that aggravate pain. For fissures that just won't heal—or chronic fissures—surgical options are available.

Bowel Obstructions and Fecal Impactions

When constipation is severe enough such that stool is sitting around in the colon for prolonged periods of time, it can become so dried out and hardened that it forms a plug. The plug forms a blockage so that the colon cannot pass any stool no matter how much it contracts, and waste begins backing up. This is referred to as a **fecal impaction**. Fecal impactions are typically painful—especially after eating—and can even result in vomiting.

Sometimes people with fecal impactions will use lots of laxatives to try to alleviate their constipation, and these laxatives draw water into the colon. If you're lucky, the force of this fluid will dislodge the impacted stool. Often, however, the dried-up stool plug remains stubbornly in place. The fluid that's been drawn into the colon from laxative use will continue to build pressure until it leaks around the edges of the stool plug and forces its way out in a dramatic, watery exit called **overflow diarrhea**. Overflow diarrhea can often result in **fecal incontinence** (pooping accidents or inability to hold in your stool) since it is so liquid, forceful, and hard to hold in. If impacted stool cannot be dislodged at home through laxatives or manual maneuvers, it may require hospitalization to get the job done. People who are impacted (or suspect that they are) should *not* eat lots of fiber in an attempt to remedy the problem, as it will just add more residue to a clogged-up pipeline.

Electrolyte Deficiencies

When diarrhea is severe or prolonged, it can result in excess losses of important minerals called electrolytes—namely, sodium, potassium, chloride, and/or magnesium. Electrolytes play a key role in keeping you hydrated, and they also act as important electrical conductors for muscle contractions—including your heart's regular beating. In other words, replenishing electrolytes is an important consideration if you're losing a lot of fluid from diarrhea.

Alarm Symptoms

If you experience any of the following symptoms with or without diarrhea or constipation, you should promptly consult your doctor or a gastroenterologist to be checked out.

- **Blood in your stool**—which may appear bright red or black, depending on its point of origin
- **White or gray-colored stools**
- **Unintentional weight loss of more than a few pounds**
- **Fever accompanying a change in your bowel patterns**
- **Nausea or vomiting associated with your diarrhea or constipation**
- **Dehydration**—which may present as excessive thirst, fatigue, headaches, decreased urination, dark yellow urine, dizziness, dry skin
- **Debilitating abdominal or anal pain**

Lastly, see a doctor if you find yourself being awakened overnight with the need to have a bowel movement. While this is not necessarily an alarm symptom, it's still not normal and should prompt a visit to a gastroenterologist.

The Mechanics
of Digestive Transit

*How Food and Waste Move Through
You, and What Affects Their Speed*

IN ORDER TO UNDERSTAND WHAT'S gone awry when things are amiss in the bathroom—and how best to respond to it—you first need to understand how your digestive tract is *supposed* to function. So before delving into the details of all the ways your gut can be dysfunctional, let's start with a brief tour through a well-functioning digestive system, following a mouthful of food from first bite until whatever remains of it exits out the proverbial back door.

The First Leg of the Journey:
The Upper Gastrointestinal Tract

The esophagus (food pipe) and stomach are the first two organs of the **gastrointestinal** tract, and collectively they are often referred to as the upper GI tract. Once you chew and swallow your food, it enters into the stomach, whose role is to blenderize it into enough of a liquid consistency that it can be squirted out a tiny muscular opening on the bottom called the **pylorus**. While activity in the upper GI tract typically has little bearing on what happens for you later on in the bathroom, I'll address a few of the possible scenarios in which diarrhea in particular can have its root this early in the digestive process.

There is a digestive system nerve-signaling reflex that partly originates in the stomach that does play a role in triggering forward motion (peristalsis) in the colon—a neighborhood of the digestive tract that is separated from the stomach by about ten to sixteen feet of small intestine lying between them. This nerve reflex is called the **gastrocolic reflex**, or GCR. The GCR is a mechanism that enables the far upstream part of the digestive tract to communicate with the far downstream part of the digestive tract, essentially giving it a heads-up that a meal is coming down the pipeline. Since the abdominal cavity only has so much room, after all, when more matter comes in, it can be helpful to move some matter out. When nerve receptors perceive stretch of the stomach walls in response to eating, they trigger this nerve reflex; moreover, a greater stretch from a larger-volume meal is more likely to trigger the GCR than a minimal stretch from a few small bites of something. The GCR is why we are more likely to poop soon after a meal, especially a larger meal. (As an aside, the arrival of fat in the early part of the small intestine can also trigger the GCR, which is why rich, oily, or fatty meals can also trigger a bowel movement soon after eating.)

While the GCR is a completely normal nerve reflex, many people with diarrhea-predominant irritable bowel syndrome (IBS-D; Chapter 4) have a highly sensitive, exaggerated gastrocolic reflex that can overcommunicate a message of **motility** to the colon. Whereas someone without IBS might eat a large, bulky salad for lunch and then have a gentle urge to move their bowels about an hour or so later, it's not uncommon for someone with IBS-D to eat a salad and find themselves running to the bathroom with urgent, crampy diarrhea within fifteen minutes or so. It's as if the colon interprets the GCR as a five-alarm fire and starts spasming in a race to free up room for what it thinks must be the mother-of-all-meals. This is caused by a dysfunctional communication channel between the brain and the intestines (called the **brain-gut axis**), where the brain routinely overinterprets stimuli it receives from the gut and sends back inappropriately heightened responses to a variety of common gut passers-through, like large meals, higher-fat foods, coffee, spices, or alcohol.

Another way in which diarrhea can be attributed to issues that originate in the stomach is if the stomach is emptying food too rapidly into the intestines rather than squirting it out a little bit at a time. This most commonly occurs in people who have had surgeries on their stomachs in which the pylorus has been removed, including certain weight loss surgeries or in surgical resections for stomach cancer. It can also happen if the pylorus just isn't functioning properly. When large volumes of food enter the small intestine rapidly, it is called **dumping** and will result in a type of osmotic diarrhea similar to what I describe in Chapter 5 that I've nicknamed the "sugar runs." When people experience dumping, it is usually high-carbohydrate and high-sugar foods—and especially sugary beverages—that trigger the worst symptoms.

The Journey Through Your Small Intestine

Still, with these few notable exceptions, diarrhea usually originates with problems in either the small intestine or the colon (large intestine)—or problems originating elsewhere that affect how food and nutrients are absorbed in the intestines. Constipation, in contrast, typically has its roots in the colon—or problems originating elsewhere that affect motility or function of the colon. To lay the groundwork for the explanations that follow in the remaining chapters of this book, it's important to understand some basics about your intestines' structures and functions.

The small intestine is divided into three neighborhoods: the duodenum, the jejunum, and the ileum, as depicted in Figure 2-1. Collectively, these segments are where the vast majority of digestion and nutrient absorption takes place: Food is broken down by a variety of enzymes into its component building blocks, and whatever can be absorbed into the body will be taken up by the cells lining the small intestine and distributed to cells throughout the body through the bloodstream. Different nutrients are absorbed

24

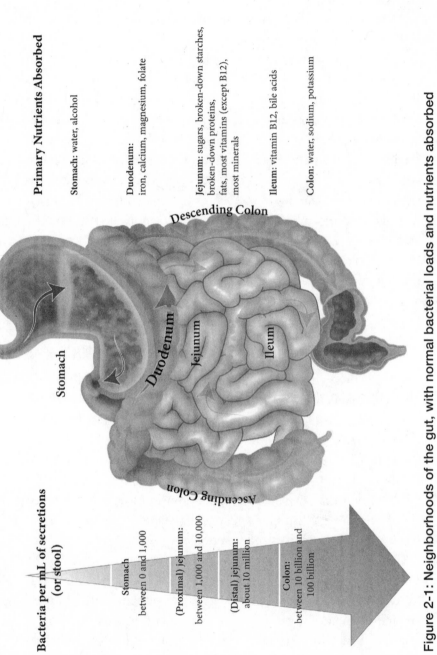

Figure 2-1: Neighborhoods of the gut, with normal bacterial loads and nutrients absorbed
Artwork by Mehtonen Medical Studios

in different segments of the small intestine, as Figure 2-1 shows. Starches and sugars are broken down and absorbed early on in the digestive process in the duodenum, first by enzymes from the pancreas, such as amylase, but mostly thanks to a series of digestive enzymes known as **disaccharidases** that are manufactured on the spot by the cells that line the small intestine. The rapid absorbability of starches and sugars is precisely why these foods can have such an immediate effect on your blood sugar. Examples of disaccharidase enzymes include lactase, maltase, and sucrase-isomaltase, and I discuss these more in Chapters 5 and 13. Special receptors for fructose sugars that line this segment of the small intestine finish off some of the additional sugar-digesting work that the pancreatic enzymes and disaccharidases don't handle.

As the mushed-up meal proceeds through the small intestine, proteins and fats are broken down (digested) by enzymes, and digestive fluids made by the pancreas and liver are delivered into the intestine in response to eating. The main enzymes made by the pancreas are **amylase** (digests certain carbohydrates), **proteases** (digest certain proteins), and **lipase** (digests fats). These are discussed more in Chapter 6 in the section on pancreatic insufficiency, where inadequate production of these enzymes can cause a type of diarrhea. In addition, the liver makes a digestive fluid called **bile**, which aids in the digestion of fat by emulsifying large fat globules into smaller fat globules, essentially exposing more of the fat to the digesting action of lipase. Bile is injected into the intestines directly from the liver and from storage in the gallbladder in response to eating, meaning that even people who have had their gallbladder removed have a backup system to ensure bile is provided to help with fat digestion. When digestion is complete, bile is broken down into its component parts—some of which are called **bile acids**. Bile acids are recycled at the tail end of the ileum, which means they are absorbed back into the intestinal cells and sent to the liver via the bloodstream so that the liver can manufacture more bile. When this recycling process works well, it's mighty efficient! When it doesn't, you might experience a type of diarrhea described in Chapter 6 in the section on bile acid malabsorption.

PANCREATIC ENZYMES NEVER FORGET

Patients often ask me if the body loses the ability to digest certain foods if they haven't eaten them for a long time. Specifically, vegetarians wonder whether they can digest meat again if they've abstained for years, and people who have followed gluten-free diets by choice (not because of celiac disease) similarly wonder if their guts can handle gluten again after all that time apart.

In fact, our body's protein-digesting enzymes are not specific to individual foods: We do not have separate protein-digesting enzymes for meat versus beans versus gluten. Our bodies release a set of general protein-digesting enzymes (proteases) in response to eating anything—regardless of whether it even contains protein—and these enzymes work by targeting specific bonds that hold protein chains together and breaking them apart. Whether these bonds are in meat, nuts, gluten, or any other protein doesn't matter!

As we progress deeper and deeper into the digestive tract, from duodenum to jejunum to ileum, you'll notice from Figure 2-1 that the number of bacteria hanging around increases exponentially. Still, even in the lower reaches of the small bowel—the ileum, right next to the colon—the load of bacteria pales in comparison with that found in the colon. This is very much by design. It would be quite problematic if we were to harbor loads and loads of bacteria in the early sections of our small intestine when there was still so much yet-to-be-digested food passing through. After all, bacteria love to eat (technically, ferment) many of the same foods that we do—especially certain sugars and carbs—and when they are presented with a buffet of these, they will compete with you for the meal. The process can create a lot of painful gas and bloating. Too many bacteria in the small intestine can also impair the recyclability of those bile acids by modifying them in a way that renders them less re-absorbable in the ileum. This, too, is a reason that people might experience (bile acid) diarrhea when they overgrow bacteria in the small intestine (see Chapter 6 on SIBO).

The Final Leg of the
Digestive Journey: The Colon

The colon is also known as your large intestine, and it starts off with a short little segment called the cecum and ends with a short segment called the **rectum**. At five feet long, the colon is much shorter than the small intestine, but typically undigested food (now waste) still spends more time traveling through it. The average transit time of a solid meal through the length of the small intestine is three to eight hours, whereas typical transit time through the colon is ten to forty hours. There are many, many factors that affect transit time of waste through the colon. In Chapter 4 on functional GI disorders like diarrhea-predominant irritable bowel syndrome (IBS-D), I discuss the role of gut hormones on the pace of colonic motility, as well as that of a neurotransmitter, or nerve-signaling molecule, called **serotonin**. (In fact, medications that either enhance or block serotonin receptors in the gut are commonly used to treat IBS with constipation or IBS with diarrhea, respectively.) Thyroid hormones also play a role in gut motility; in fact, hypothyroidism—or low thyroid hormone levels—is one possible cause of constipation. The composition of your diet can also affect colonic transit time. For example, bulky forms of fiber can speed along colonic motility by stimulating the muscle-lined intestinal walls to contract.

There are several things going on in the colon during the digestive process that have relevance to the consistency of your stool and, in turn, your bowel regularity. The first is reabsorption of water and electrolytes from the waste stream back into the body. Undigested food exiting the small intestine is still watery mush, but by the time it leaves the large intestine in the form of a bowel movement, it's supposed to be a soft but formed (solid) stool. This magical transformation is the simple result of excess water from the waste having spent the right amount of time in the colon for its moisture content to be perfected. When stool rushes through the colon such that there is not enough time for excess water to be reabsorbed, the result will be loose, poorly formed stools—or even watery diarrhea. When stool spends too much time dragging its way through a too-slow colon, then too much moisture will be reabsorbed back into the body. The result will often be extremely hard, dried-out stools that looked like cracked sausages or emerge as hard little pebbles. Many remedies that help maintain moisture in the stool are available for people who experience these symptoms; they include stool softeners like Colace (docusate sodium) and water-binding laxatives like magnesium and PEG-3350 (Mira-LAX), all of which are described later in Chapter 9.

There are also factors that can influence the fluid content of stools apart from transit time. In cases of inflammation (Chapter 7), the cells lining the colon may be actively secreting more fluid into the intestines, making stools loose or watery. In cases of bile acid malabsorption (Chapter 6), the arrival of bile acids into the colon similarly triggers the cells of the colon to release more fluid into the waste stream, and will similarly result in a tendency toward diarrhea.

The colon is also where the vast majority of the gut microbiota—which now enjoys celebrity status—resides. The gut microbiota is a trillions-strong, highly complex ecosystem of microorganisms that is as individual to you as your fingerprints, and whose composition is highly adapted to your local environment and diet. The gut microbiota of someone in urban Tokyo who eats a reasonably fiber-rich local diet will look very different from that of someone in rural Colorado who eats a reasonably fiber-rich local diet, but trying to compare them and decide which is healthier would be like trying to determine whether a tropical rain forest is healthier than a northeastern deciduous forest. They're just different, and each can be healthy in its own context.

The thousand (or more) different species of bacteria and other organisms that make up your gut microbiome do a whole bunch of alchemy in there. They take some elements of your waste—mostly undigested fiber and whatever other nutrients escaped digestion in the small intestine—and ferment it for themselves. In the process, they create all kinds of magical products:

- For one, they can liberate some calories from fibers that are indigestible to humans; an estimated 5% to 10% of our daily energy actually derives from this process. (I know many of us weight-conscious modern humans aren't too psyched about these hidden bonus calories, but our prehistoric ancestors surely depended on them with their high-fiber diets and unreliable access to food.)

- They also manufacture some vitamins for our use as part of their metabolic activities—mostly vitamin K and some B vitamins.

- Certain types of bacteria are also known to make compounds called short-chain fatty acids (SCFAs) when fed the fibers of their choice—and these SCFAs have been credited with a variety of health-promoting contributions, most notably in helping to prevent colon cancer. **Postbiotics** is the term that has been bestowed upon SCFAs when marketed as a dietary supplement in an attempt to circumvent the whole eating fiber for "health benefits" thing and sell one of the end products of fiber fermentation directly to consumers in pill form.

- And beyond SCFAs—there are a host of other chemicals that our gut microbes produce as the result of metabolizing compounds in our waste that are thought to hold the key to many other physiological processes and outcomes—including how our microbes communicate with our brains and other cells of the body to influence pain sensation, mood, immune function, and even metabolism of energy. In fact, scientists who study the so-called **metabolome** (the collection of metabolic by-products created by the microbiome) devote their entire careers to understanding the substances that our gut microbes produce as a result of their interactions with dietary compounds we consume, and how these substances affect human health. Once these bacterial metabolites are better identified and understood, it is only a matter of time before the current global obsession with supplementing probiotics will be replaced with an equally robust effort to supplement a variety of the beneficial stuff they make instead.

This brief written trip through the digestive tract took much less time than an actual trip would, but hopefully you've brushed up on your knowledge of basic digestive functioning so that you'll be ready to dig in to the chapters ahead. While you certainly shouldn't need a medical degree to understand why you struggle with bowel regularity, it's still important for you to have a basic, correct understanding of how your body is supposed to work and in what way it might not be working properly. Many people find that their medical visits are so short and rushed that it can seem like their doctor is just throwing medication at the problem; by understanding more about your potential problem before you even step into the doctor's office, you can be a better partner in your own care by offering the most relevant information about your symptoms, and you will be better equipped to ask questions about the types of tests and treatments your doctor has at their disposal.

How to Use This Book, and a Diagnostic Quiz

THIS BOOK IS DESIGNED TO be a self-help tool, written in a choose-your-own-adventure style. Unless you're my mom or my editor, I don't expect that you'll read it cover to cover. Instead, I mean for you to read the first two chapters to help ground yourself in the basics of digestive physiology—how things work, what's considered normal, what is cause for alarm. The rest of the book is meant for you to skip around in based on the results of the quiz that follows.

I designed this quiz in collaboration with my gastroenterologist colleague Dr. Eric Goldstein as a paper version of the real-time brain algorithm that we use in our clinical practice when patients show up complaining of diarrhea, constipation, or some combo thereof. Trained clinicians typically ask a small number of key questions that quickly help us narrow down the likeliest causes of your symptoms. While the symptom of "diarrhea" may seem pretty general, your answers to the questions we ask are actually really differentiating among the many, many causes of diarrhea, and within just five minutes of pointed Q&A, we can often develop a hypothesis to road test. The same goes for constipation. Believe it or not, there are many different ways to NOT go to the bathroom!

The quiz in this chapter is meant to approximate the type of in-office detective work we do, and your scores will direct you to the chapter(s) in the book that seem most relevant to the symptoms you experience. Each column, labeled A through G, corresponds to a type of medical issue that causes bowel irregularity; there is a decoder key at the end of the quiz that explains what each letter stands for. If you read my first book, *The Bloated Belly Whisperer*, then the quiz format will be very familiar to you, and the rest of the instructions below may give you a bit of déjà vu. Read the instructions carefully before attempting the quiz; I got tons of social media pings from readers of my previous book who skipped this step and were utterly befuddled by how to complete the quiz and understand the results. Please and thank you.

One last disclaimer before you proceed: While the quiz was developed by a very experienced dietitian (me) in collaboration with a pretty brilliant gastroenterologist, we are not your personal dietitian and gastroenterologist. In other words, your results on this quiz do not constitute a definitive medical diagnosis. The results of this quiz are meant to provide an educated guess about the root of your problem based on your symptom pattern. The intent is for you to bring this educated guess with you to your own personal doctor so that you can have a productive conversation about tests or treatment trials that would confirm or rule out the suspected diagnosis. Even if you were my personal patient, as a dietitian it is not within my scope of professional practice to diagnose any medical condition. I just read the proverbial tea leaves of your symptoms as they relate to food choices to help you and your doctor narrow down the most likely possibilities so you can find inner peace faster.

Directions for Taking the Quiz

1. Read each question and identify the most fitting option(s) that best describe your bowel movement patterns and gastrointestinal symptoms. For questions that allow it, you may choose more than one answer.

2. Alongside each answer, you will find one or more empty circles. Fill in ALL THE EMPTY CIRCLES in the row alongside your chosen response. See the first sample question as an example of what that should look like.

3. For any given question, if there are no answers provided that accurately describe your experience, or if you're simply unsure of the answer, just leave it blank. Do not choose an answer that does not accurately represent your situation. Similarly, questions 4 and 5 are for people who are diarrhea prone and constipation prone, respectively. If you are not diarrhea prone, skip question 4. If you are not constipation prone, skip question 5. If you experience alternating constipation and diarrhea, then you can and should answer both.

4. When you are finished taking the quiz, count up the total number of shaded circles in each column, from A through H, and write the sum of each column in the total box at the bottom of each column.

5. Make note of which column numbers have the highest number of shaded boxes. Look for the corresponding diagnoses and chapter numbers or page numbers in the decoder key that follows the quiz. You should flip ahead to the chapter that corresponds to the diagnosis with which you scored the most symptom matches and read the

introductory paragraphs of the chapter to see if the condition description sounds familiar. Constipation-prone readers will almost certainly be directed to one of Chapters 9, 10, or 11. Diarrhea-prone readers will likely be directed to one of Chapters 4, 5, 6, 7, or 8. If you experience a mix of diarrhea and constipation, just follow along to the chapter where the quiz results lead you!

6. If your quiz results direct you to the chapter on malabsorptive diarrhea (Chapter 6), you should read the introductory paragraphs of EACH condition it contains before deciding whether one of these conditions may apply to you. There are four distinct medical conditions described in this chapter.

7. After reading your top-ranked chapter/section, if you feel that it did not accurately describe your situation, proceed to the chapter/section where you had the second-highest number of symptom matches. And so on.

8. If your symptom matches score pretty evenly across multiple chapters in both the diarrhea and constipation sections and you're not sure where to go first, you should start by reading the section on SIBO in Chapter 6, "Malabsorptive Mayhem." If the SIBO section doesn't resonate, you may need to visit the introductory paragraphs of multiple chapters you matched with to see which one strikes the closest chord.

A Note for Those Prone to *Both* Diarrhea *and* Constipation

It may be tricky to classify yourself as being diarrhea prone OR constipation prone when you tend to experience both, and it's possible that your quiz results will be somewhat muddier than those of someone who clearly fits one pattern more so than the other. For this reason, I'd like to plant some seeds for you to consider as you read through the various chapters in this book.

Sometimes diarrhea can be the result of chronic constipation. What I mean by this is that the diarrhea is really a function of underlying constipation, and once the constipation is resolved, the diarrhea disappears, too. One example of this is **overflow diarrhea**, which I described in Chapter 1. Overflow diarrhea occurs when a person has a large amount of stool backed up in the colon that has become obstructive in nature; that is, it has formed somewhat of a blockage. In this scenario, attempting to take laxatives to alleviate the constipation can result in watery diarrhea that does not actually dislodge any of the hard, dried-out stool. The diarrhea is literally the liquid that the laxatives have pulled into the bowel, and it's forcing its way around the margins of the stool blockage. If you are someone who goes many days at a time with no bowel movements and then experiences liquid-only stools when you try to use a laxative, you should consider that your main problem is actually constipation. So I'd explore Chapters 9 to 11 of this book and not bother looking for organic causes of the diarrhea.

There's another type of diarrhea that's secondary to constipation that I've nicknamed **"dam-breaking diarrhea."** We see this type of diarrhea a lot in patients with constipation-predominant IBS (IBS-C; Chapter 10). The general pattern is that you may not move your bowels for two to three days in a row (or just move tiny little dribs and drabs that barely count), and then on the fourth day, it's like the dam breaks and your bowels are suddenly emptying all four days' worth of stool over the course of a single day.

You're in and out of the bathroom several times throughout the day. The stools may start off hard or formed, but with each passing movement they get softer, softer, and softer until they eventually wind up as diarrhea. Sometimes the dam breaks because you take a laxative, or sometimes it breaks because you eat something that's known to stimulate your bowels—like a high-fat meal, a large-volume meal, or a high-lactose dessert like ice cream. And sometimes your colon will just break the dam on its own accord, as if it's following an unpublished schedule that you've not been consulted about. Once again, I treat this type of diarrhea as fundamentally a product of underlying constipation and would direct you to Chapters 9 and 10 to start with, though I've had chronically constipated patients whose dam-breaking diarrhea was actually triggered by sugar intolerances (osmotic diarrhea) like those described in Chapter 5. See the case study at the end of that chapter for a real-life example of how this may present itself.

A Note for Those Whose Bowel Problems Started After Infection with COVID-19

Some cases of COVID-19 affect the gastrointestinal tract, causing symptoms from nausea and vomiting to abdominal pain and diarrhea. If the aftermath of your COVID infection is the origin story of your ongoing, persistent digestive complaints, there may be a few chapters in this book with relevance for you. If you are diarrhea prone since having COVID-19, the section in Chapter 4 that describes post-infectious IBS may be most relevant to you. However, if you are a COVID-19 "long-hauler" experiencing a constellation of symptoms related to impaired nervous system function (a diagnosis called dysautonomia), you may actually find yourself more constipation prone. In this case, the advice shared in Chapter 10 may be the most relevant to your situation.

THE REGULAR QUIZ

SAMPLE QUESTION: DO NOT COUNT Coffee has the following effect on my bowels:	A	B	C	D	E	F	G	H
Stimulates a welcome, helpful nudge to move my bowels					O	O	O	
Overstimulates my bowels in an unwelcome way (diarrhea, urgent, too-frequent bowel movements)	●			●				
Causes cramping/discomfort and does not make me go to the bathroom				O				O
Has no observable effect on my bowels (e.g., things would be about the same whether I drank it or not)	O	O		O			O	O
1. Choose all that apply: My bowel patterns most closely resemble . . .	A	B	C	D	E	F	G	H
Chronically loose stools	O	O	O	O	O			
Bowel movements are too frequent and/or too urgent	O	O	O	O	O			O
Stools are chronically hard and/or infrequent						O	O	O
Stools feel incomplete, and I need to strain even when they're soft								O
Cycle of several days constipation followed by a day with constant/multiple bowel movements or diarrhea						O	O	
I have several-day stretches of time with normal/formed stools, punctuated by random episodes of diarrhea		O		O				
2. Choose all that apply: The consistency of my stools can be described as . . .	A	B	C	D	E	F	G	H
Hard little balls						O	O	O
Lumpy, cracked sausages						O	O	O
Start off hard/dry but then get smoother, softer, or looser						O	O	O
Sticky, tarry, "toothpaste-like," hard to wipe clean		O	O					
Skinny and long, "pencil-like"								O
Loose and fluffy; disintegrates into a cloud when flushed	O	O	O					
Light colored, orangey		O	O	O				
Totally soft and unformed—like cow patties or soft-serve ice cream	O	O	O	O				
Watery		O		O	O			

(continues)

38

REGULAR

(continued)

3. Do you wake overnight with the need to have a bowel movement? (pick one)	A	B	C	D	E	F	G	H
Yes, at least once per month		O	O	O				
No	O				O	O	O	O
Very infrequently, but it does happen occasionally		O		O				

4. If you are diarrhea prone, the foods most likely to trigger symptoms are (check all that apply)	A	B	C	D	E	F	G	H
Milk or ice cream	O	O	O	O				
Entrée-sized salad with olive oil, no vinegar	O			O				
Turkey sandwich on bread or plain pasta (no sauce)	O		O					
Starchy gluten-free foods like rice, potatoes, or bananas		O						
Fermented foods like cheese, red wine, soy sauce, or salami					O			
Fried foods	O		O	O				
Candy, juice, or other low-fat sweets		O		O				
Tomato sauce	O	O			O			
Fruit	O	O		O				
I have never been able to connect my diarrhea to specific foods or categories of food		O	O	O	O			
Regardless of what I eat, I always need to defecate within 15–30 minutes after eating	O			O				

5. If you are constipation prone, what happens when you try laxative medications?	A	B	C	D	E	F	G	H
Laxative medications improve my stool form and/or help me go more frequently				O		O	O	
Laxative medications at low doses do nothing; high doses just give me watery diarrhea							O	O
Laxatives help me go more frequently, but my stools still never feel complete and/or I strain to pass even soft stools							O	O

6. Choose one: Eating high "roughage" foods like salads, berries, nuts, or popcorn generally make my bowel patterns . . .	A	B	C	D	E	F	G	H
Better						O	O	
Worse	O			O				O
I don't know/no noticeable difference/can go either way		O	O		O		O	

7. If you have taken a fiber supplement (e.g., psyllium/Metamucil, Benefiber, Citrucel) in the past, what was its effect?	A	B	C	D	E	F	G	H
Helped regulate/improve my bowel movements	O					O	O	
Made me feel worse by causing me to move my bowels TOO much	O			O				
Made me feel bloated/heavy and did not help regulate my bowel movements							O	O
Did not seem to make a noticeable difference for me		O	O		O			O
8. In terms of digestive symptoms, mornings are generally . . .	A	B	C	D	E	F	G	H
My best time of the day				O		O	O	
My worst time of the day	O							
Neither best nor worst consistently; may depend how I felt at bedtime the previous evening		O	O		O		O	O
9. In addition to my defecation problems, I also have the following symptoms (check all that apply)	A	B	C	D	E	F	G	H
A visibly distended belly that starts the day a little bloated and builds as the day progresses						O	O	O
Unintended weight loss			O	O				
Unexplained iron deficiency			O	O				
Nausea or early satiety (feeling full after only eating a small amount)					O		O	O
Hives, rashes, or chronic itching					O			
Extreme amounts of bowel gas (farting) every night no matter what I eat			O	O			O	O
Episodes of bowel gas/farting that seem to be better/worse depending on what I eat	O	O		O	O	O		
History of low vitamin B12 levels even though I am not vegetarian/vegan			O	O				
New onset food intolerances (foods I used to eat regularly now cause digestive distress)	O	O		O				
Pain in my anus or rectum				O				O
Somewhat regular rectal bleeding/blood in my stool				O				

(continues)

(continued)

10. If you experience abdominal pain regularly . . .	A	B	C	D	E	F	G	H
It is improved or alleviated after I have a bowel movement	O						O	
It is not improved or alleviated after I have a bowel movement			O	O				
It may be worse after I have a bowel movement								O
11. If you have ever tried to follow a low-carb diet (avoiding grains, sugar, fruits, beans, etc.), how did it affect your bowel movements?	A	B	C	D	E	F	G	H
It made my bowel movements better/more regular		O		O		O		
It made my bowel movements worse/less regular	O		O	O		O	O	O
No noticeable effect on my bowel movements			O		O			O

TOTALS ⇨								
	A	B	C	D	E	F	G	H

Scoring the REGULAR Quiz

If you scored the most matches with column . . .	. . . your symptoms most closely resemble this diagnosis/these diagnoses . . .	. . . so start on this chapter/page
A	Diarrhea-predominant irritable bowel syndrome (IBS-D)	Chapter 4/p. 43
B	Osmotic diarrhea from sugar intolerance: sucrose, maltose, fructose, lactose, and/or polyols	Chapter 5/p. 81
C	Malabsorptive diarrhea from one or more of the following: bile acid malabsorption, small intestinal bacterial overgrowth (SIBO), celiac disease, pancreatic insufficiency	Chapter 6/p. 97
D	Inflammatory bowel disease	Chapter 7/p. 133
E	Histamine intolerance	Chapter 8/p. 167
F	Constipation due to inadequate fiber intake	Chapter 9/p. 195
G	Constipation-predominant irritable bowel syndrome (IBS-C)	Chapter 10/p. 207
H	Constipation due to outlet dysfunction	Chapter 11/p. 223

PART II

Fast and Loose

The Many Kinds of Diarrhea

Functional Gastrointestinal Disorders

Irritable Bowel Syndrome (IBS-D)

IRRITABLE BOWEL SYNDROME (IBS) HAS got to be one of the most misunderstood conditions I encounter. Some patients are under the impression that it's a "last resort" diagnosis—dispensed only when doctors can't find evidence of anything else to explain your symptoms, which may include frequent, often crampy, and loose bowel movements that tend to cluster in the morning; regular bouts of abdominal pain that are usually relieved on defecation; irregular cycles of defecation in which you may not have the urge to move your bowels for two to three days at a time, followed by an all-day toileting marathon in which your body seems to be making up for lost time; or the sudden, urgent need to defecate, especially following meals, after eating "roughage" or high-fat foods, or in stressful situations. In other words, my patients are often given the impression that they are labeled as having IBS when their doctor can't find something "real" wrong with them. It is also common for patients to be given the impression that their IBS is a psychological disorder; that somehow they are causing their own symptoms due to stress or anxiety, and that, therefore, their digestive symptoms are "all in their head."

In my experience, these pervasive myths about IBS often contribute to stigma and unnecessarily compromised quality of life for patients with the condition. Laboring under the (mis)belief that IBS isn't a real disorder, patients may be unaware of the many interventions available for symptom management. Being told that the condition is all in your head and prescribed an antidepressant medication without an explanation can increase stigma around the condition and can similarly interfere with a patient's willingness to pursue treatment. Prior to landing in my office, many of my patients who have lived with IBS-D for years—if not decades—have completely contorted their lives to work around their unpredictable bowel behavior. They cancel vacations or back out of social situations when there are concerns about bathroom access; they change jobs to create work schedules that don't demand early-morning arrival times; they abstain from eating on days they have to be out and about for appointments or travel so that the risk of having an attack of diarrhea is minimized.

But understanding some of the mechanisms that underpin IBS-D can help you modify your diet to prevent provoking symptoms, and understanding the many available medical remedies and behavioral therapies available can address whatever gaps in symptom control that diet alone can't remedy. IBS may not yet be curable, but that certainly doesn't mean you just have to live with its symptoms.

Diarrhea-Predominant Irritable Bowel Syndrome (IBS-D)

Irritable bowel syndrome (IBS) in all its forms is known as a **functional gastrointestinal disorder (FGID)**—or, by the preferred emerging term, a **disorder of the gut-brain interaction (DGBI)**. The qualifier "functional" refers to the fact that while the bowel may not be behaving normally, there is no visible structural or objectively measurable cause for this dysfunction. For example, you may experience diarrhea several days per week, but a **colonoscopy** shows that the colon's tissues are perfectly intact and healthy looking—with no inflammation in sight. You may be prone to debilitating abdominal pain, but imaging studies of your abdomen—like ultrasounds or CT scans—don't show any abnormalities in the digestive system organs or abdominal cavity that would account for the degree of pain you experience. You may experience diarrhea, pain, or abdominal bloating associated with certain foods—but blood antibody tests for food allergy and celiac disease all come back negative.

This is because the symptoms of IBS are caused by factors that remain largely invisible to us, at least in a clinical setting. Namely, the symptoms of IBS result from a disruption of the normal motility (movement-related) and sensory (sensation-related) processes of the gut, and these disruptions are largely related to abnormal activity of chemical messengers like **hormones** and nerve-signaling messengers called **neurotransmitters**.

For example, available research suggests that people with IBS may have abnormally overactive responses of a gut hormone called cholecystokinin (CCK), which is secreted after fat-containing meals. Levels of another gut hormone called vasoactive intestinal peptide (VIP) are also found to be higher in people with IBS compared with healthy controls. Since VIP stimulates bowel motility, it seems likely that higher concentrations of it could help account for the characteristically loose stools and urgent, crampy diarrhea that people with IBS-D experience. Unfortunately, doctors can't really visualize or measure these hormone levels in a clinical setting.

A neurotransmitter called **serotonin**, which is referred to as 5-HT (for 5-hydroxytryptamine) in the biz, also plays a key role in IBS-D symptoms. Serotonin is produced and released by specialized cells that line our gut, and it plays a key role in communicating information about what's happening in the gut to our brain. It does so by attaching to serotonin receptors on nerve endings that line the intestinal wall. As a result of its communication with the brain, serotonin plays a key role in gut motility, secretions, and pain perception. However, it's been observed that the brains of people with IBS tend to respond inappropriately to messages sent up by serotonin. A distress signal sent by the gut to the brain in response to gaseous distension *should* be met with a calming, reassuring, pain-suppressing reaction, but in IBS the brain may interpret the signals with heightened pain and alarmist hypermotility messages. As such, medications that block certain of these serotonin receptors in the gut, including low doses of antidepressant medications, have been shown to reduce pain and diarrhea in people with IBS-D.

As the paragraphs above describe, abnormal gut hormone levels or GI tract reactivity is a key contributor to diarrhea in many people with IBS-D, as are abnormal brain responses to nerve signals originating from the gut—both of which affect the colon's motility and secretions. When the brain sends chemical messengers to signal the colon to speed up its motility in response to a nonemergency situation, the resulting hypermotility leaves too little time for excess water in the stool to be reabsorbed back into the body, and we get loose or watery stools.

Treatments for IBS-D, therefore, are often targeted at various aspects of this dysfunction; they are described in greater detail later in this chapter. Soluble fiber, for example, helps absorb some of this excess water while slowing down the stool's transit time through the colon. Medications such as tricyclic antidepressants (TCAs) can help reduce diarrhea by rebalancing the relative levels of various neurotransmitters in the gut and possibly also by blocking the action of histamine; note that these meds are acting directly on the gut to affect motility and are *not* prescribed under the presumption that a psychological condition like depression or anxiety is the cause of IBS symptoms. (Typically, the dose of a TCA that a gastroenterologist would prescribe is a fraction of what a psychiatrist would prescribe for depression.) A variety of other medications that act directly on the colon to counteract motility or muscle spasms are effective to help chill out the hyperreactive colon and prevent urgency or too-frequent urges to defecate.

But any discussion of IBS-D would be incomplete without mentioning the thing that separates IBS from any old case of rapid gut transit time: over-sensation of pain to stimuli within the gut that's referred to as **visceral hypersensitivity**. One of my gastroenterologist colleagues explains visceral hypersensitivity by using the analogy of having an internal pain thermostat that's turned up too high. Two people may have the same amount of gas in their intestines, but the person with IBS is more likely to experience the pressure within the bowel produced by this normal amount of gas as extremely uncomfortable—or downright painful—than the person without IBS. While IBS symptoms are not all in your head, this aspect of IBS can accurately be said to be in your brain. That is, it results from how your brain interprets—or overinterprets—stimuli within the gut, whether those stimuli are distension from gas or stool or sensations from chemical irritants like alcohol or spicy food. Some treatments for abdominal pain associated with IBS-D, therefore, are aimed at turning down the pain thermostat by modifying the hormones or nerve signals that facilitate communication between the gut and brain; they are described in more detail later in this chapter.

How Do Symptoms of IBS-D Present?

There are some very common symptom patterns associated with IBS-D. For starters, mornings are usually the most symptomatic time of day. This seems to be related to natural peaks in the hormone cortisol, a stress hormone whose job it is to wake up the gut from overnight sleep mode. Cortisol levels start rising at 4 a.m. and peak by 10 a.m., during which time our bowels are primed to poop; think of mornings as a biological window of poop-ortunity. Piling on any additional stimuli—a few sips of coffee, a few bites of breakfast—is often enough to stimulate a bowel movement for anyone. But when you have IBS-D, the bowel is hyperreactive to these normal stimuli—coffee especially. The first morning bowel movement may be somewhat normal in appearance, but it often sets off a series of spasms that result in sudden-onset, crampy, repeat trips back to the bathroom. A second bowel movement quickly follows the first, and often there may be a third, a fourth, or even more over the course of a brief period of time in the morning. It's common for stools to become looser and looser as the morning progresses. Many people find they can't reliably make it out of the house in time for work or other morning appointments due to this series of constant urges to defecate. It's common for people with IBS-D to wake up an hour or more earlier than they need to just to get a head start on the toileting marathon so they can be finished in time to leave the house for work. For people with IBS-D, morning symptoms may be especially severe if they consumed alcohol the previous night, or had a particularly large, high-fat, or late dinner.

While mornings are typically active symptom-wise for people with IBS-D, there are some common symptom patterns that can strike later in the day, too. Any meal that provokes significant stomach stretch—whether a large-size lunch salad or sizable portion of cooked food—can trigger a bowel spasm within minutes that results in an urgent need to poop. This bowel movement may be formed or can be diarrhea—leading to the common impression among my patients with IBS-D that "salad goes right through me." (In fact, it's not the salad you just ate that you're pooping out fifteen minutes later; rather, it's the salad you just ate that's provoking a forceful wave of motility in your colon, which has you pooping out last night's dinner somewhat urgently.) Similarly, higher-fat meals can provoke this sudden-onset, urgent need to defecate. As you may recall from Chapter 2, the normal nerve reflex that results in the colon's forward motility following a meal is called the **gastrocolic reflex**; people with IBS-D are said to have an accelerated or exaggerated gastrocolic reflex. In other words, the gut's hair-trigger sensory thermostat overreacts to the stimulation of an ever-so-slightly larger or fattier meal and sends you running to the bathroom.

People with IBS typically do not wake overnight with the need to move their bowels, and it's not common to lose weight as the result of IBS . . . unless your symptoms have led you to severely restrict your food intake in order to avoid provoking an attack. Because IBS is not caused by malabsorption, nutritional deficiencies are not typically associated with IBS unless, once again, you restrict your diet severely in an attempt to manage your symptoms. Foods that commonly trigger diarrhea or loose, urgent bowel movements among people with IBS-D include coffee (including decaf); alcohol; fried food or other oily/fatty foods; restaurant meals in general (typically owing to the higher fat content or larger portions); dairy foods, especially higher-fat ones like ice cream or cream-based sauces; spicy foods; and large salads or other forms of "roughage" like corn, popcorn, nuts/seeds, cabbage, kale, and thick-skinned, unpeeled fruits and veggies.

Diagnosing IBS-D

According to the latest diagnostic guidelines for IBS, your doctor will first need to rule out two other main causes of diarrhea: inflammatory bowel disease (Chapter 7) and celiac disease (Chapter 6). This diagnostic workup typically involves a blood test and possibly a stool test as well. In the past, IBS was considered a diagnosis of exclusion, and patients would commonly be subjected to an extensive battery of tests: imaging studies like ultrasounds, X-rays, or abdominal CT scans; colonoscopy; and an upper endoscopy as well. Once these other causes of chronic diarrhea had been ruled out, your doctor would compare your symptom patterns against the established, symptom-based diagnostic criteria for IBS to make the diagnosis. But this exhausting and expensive approach is changing, and as the more recent guidelines described above demonstrate, doctors are increasingly encouraged to make a positive diagnosis of IBS based on symptom patterns once celiac disease and Crohn's disease have been ruled out on the basis of relatively noninvasive stool and blood tests.

In this way, IBS is a clinical diagnosis: it is made by a doctor based on observations of your reported symptoms rather than based on conclusive findings from lab test results. (There is only one scientifically validated set of biomarkers to aid in the diagnosis of IBS, and their applicability is limited to a very specific type of IBS that has an onset following an acute gastrointestinal infection and represents a minority of cases; see the discussion below about post-infectious

IBS for more details.) The diagnostic criteria for IBS—and all functional gastrointestinal disorders—are established by the Rome Foundation and are periodically updated to reflect the latest scientific evidence. The so-called **Rome Criteria** for IBS diagnosis are currently in their fourth iteration and are as follows (paraphrased):

Abdominal pain one or more times per week in the past three months, with *at least two* of the following additional symptoms:

- Pain related to defecation (pooping makes it better or worse)
- There is also a change in stool frequency
- There is also a change in stool form (appearance)

Source: Adapted from the Rome IV Criteria for the Diagnosis of IBS

DIAGNOSING POST-INFECTIOUS IBS (IBS-PI)

Some people with IBS-D report having a history of a "sensitive stomach" since childhood—which, more accurately, should be described as a "sensitive bowel," since it's not the stomach that's misbehaving in IBS. In these cases, digestive symptoms may be relatively better or relatively worse at different stages of their lives, but they've been around for a very long time. But another path to IBS-D lies in the aftermath of an acute gastrointestinal infection of some sort. A common scenario involves a perfectly healthy, gut-of-steel-type person acquiring a case of food poisoning or other form of bacterial gastroenteritis, most commonly an infection by *Campylobacter* bacteria, or picking up an intestinal parasite such as *Giardia* somewhere in their travels. People who are infected with some of the COVID-19 variants may similarly experience gastrointestinal symptoms, including diarrhea. After surviving the acute, short-lived diarrheal illness, things are never quite the same for them again digestively and they develop IBS-like symptoms. This is called **post-infectious IBS (IBS-PI)**.

One of the underlying mechanisms of IBS-PI is thought to be immune system activation that results from a temporary increase in intestinal permeability (leakiness) in the aftermath of certain bacterial infections caused by a specific toxin these bacteria produce, and/or changes in the motility patterns of the digestive tract related to the actions of the infectious agent. During an infection, the body produces antibodies against the infectious invader; these antibodies can attack the body's own tissues if molecules on those tissues resemble the original offender. When this happens, tissue damage can occur. If the damaged tissue involves the nerves, muscles, or cells lining the gut, diarrhea and/or pain can result.

There is actually a blood test called the ibs-smart test that may help your doctor identify whether your chronic diarrhea is likely to be caused by IBS-PI from common bacteria implicated in food poisoning. It measures two specific biomarkers via a blood test: anti-vinculin antibodies and anti-CdtB antibodies. In the United States, the blood test is offered by a company called Gemelli Biotech; a positive result can help support an IBS-PI diagnosis quickly, potentially allowing your doctor to bypass an extensive search for other causes. This test has been validated only for IBS-PI caused by certain bacterial infections, not from COVID-19 or other viral infections.

If you've undergone an exhaustive (and exhausting) testing process, your gastroenterologist may say something like "Good news! It's just IBS!" and it's likely to make your blood boil. What I *think* they mean by this comment is that they have ruled out a potentially life-threatening disease like colon cancer or inflammatory diseases that can lead to serious, long-term health complications like Crohn's disease (Chapter 7). True, it is objectively good news that the cause of your diarrhea and pain is not potentially life-threatening. But reflecting on the words *"just* IBS," it's not hard to understand why so many patients feel that their suffering is being dismissed. It's as if the goal of the diagnostic process was to reveal an answer about the cause of your symptoms—not to actually help improve your symptoms. You may not be dying or at risk for serious health complications—but the assault on your quality of life remains unchanged. You're still a slave to the toilet, afraid to eat at restaurants or at parties, and subject to frequent attacks of debilitating pain and anxiety-provoking, out-of-the-blue attacks of diarrhea. I wish that more doctors would use the diagnosis of IBS as a conversation starter, not a conversation ender. Once your doctor has landed on IBS as the cause of your diarrhea, we'd like this diagnostic reveal to be chased with the following sentence: "So now that we're confident that this is IBS we're dealing with here, let's talk about how we're going to manage your symptoms."

Treating IBS-D

There is no cure for irritable bowel syndrome, but there are plenty of evidence-based ways to manage its symptoms and vastly improve your quality of life.

Dietary Approaches for Managing IBS-D

Survey data reveal that the vast majority of people with IBS-D find their symptoms to be associated with specific food triggers. But there is a lot of variability in terms of what those triggers are. Therefore, I avoid dogmatic, cookie-cutter, highly restrictive diet protocols and encourage my patients to tailor their diet to their own individual symptom patterns and tolerances. For example, one common default recommendation you've likely encountered (either online, from a well-meaning medical doctor or nutritionist, or from a functional medicine practitioner or naturopath) is the importance of a gluten-free and dairy-free diet when you have IBS. Having counseled thousands of IBS patients over the past decade, I can say that while there are certainly many people with IBS-D who feel far better on gluten-free diets, there are also many others who find that a plain bagel—in all its gluten-containing glory—is their safest food on a bad digestion day. And some others come to me *thinking* they are sensitive to gluten, only to discover through our work together that they can actually handle certain (less gas-forming) types of gluten-containing foods—like sourdough bread or spelt flour–based products—just fine. **Gluten-free diets should not be a default recommendation across the board for everyone with IBS-D!** Along these same lines, some patients find that they need to avoid all dairy in order to keep their symptoms stable, while others can handle lower-fat and lactose-free dairy foods just fine.

And even beyond the highly contested world of gluten and dairy, I also encourage my patients not to get stuck in internet dogma surrounding other foods, either. Raw vegetables or greens are a great example. A kale salad might be a killer of a trigger for your IBS-D, but if you put that kale into a blender and make it into a smoothie, you can handle it just fine. In other words, forget what you've read online. There is not one single "IBS diet."

Soluble Fiber Therapy

There are a few dietary approaches I use when helping my patients with IBS-D figure out how to eat to best control their symptoms, and they are not mutually exclusive. One approach is called **soluble fiber therapy**, in which we modify the relative amounts of two different types of fiber in a person's diet to help regulate the form and transit time of bowel movements, which typically helps reduce urgency and frequency. It often involves taking a soluble fiber supplement at night before bed; reducing the amount of "roughage" (insoluble fiber) in the diet; and increasing the amount of soluble fiber from foods in the daily diet. Since soluble fiber slows down transit time through the colon and absorbs excess water while insoluble fiber speeds up transit time through the colon and doesn't hold onto any water, you can see how changing the relative amounts of these two fibers in your diet can affect your bowel movements. Chapter 12 describes this approach in great detail, with explanations for how to use a fiber supplement to manage diarrhea, and sample menus for a soluble fiber–rich day.

Portion Control

Another factor to consider in managing symptoms of IBS-D is your meal size and its fat content. With the understanding that having a hair-trigger gastrocolic reflex is typical in IBS-D, you can avoid overstimulating the gastrocolic reflex by eating **smaller meals more frequently instead of two or three larger-volume meals per day**. You can also avoid eating too much fat in a given meal or snack. I'll concede that "too much fat" is a very subjective term—what is too much for one person with IBS may be tolerated by someone else— and there are no objective guidelines I can offer with regard to the magic number of fat grams per meal that will guarantee tolerance. It may take some trial and error to figure out what amount of fat you can get away with in a sitting. High-fat foods that commonly trigger many of my patients with IBS include fried foods, cream sauces, greasy/oily takeout, ice cream, macaroni and cheese, more than one slice of pizza, steakhouse dinners, cheeseburger deluxe meals, and coconut milk–based curry dishes . . . to name but a few.

It is also worthwhile examining whether certain poorly digested sugars may be drawing excess water into the bowel and having a laxative effect, thereby worsening your stool consistency and increasing your frequency of bowel movements. Small sugar particles like lactose, fructose, or even **sucrose** (table sugar) can attract water into the colon through osmosis (remember that from eighth-grade biology class?) if they are not fully digested and absorbed in the small intestine. Similarly, several families of poorly digested sugar alcohols (also called polyols) can have this effect. Sugar alcohols both occur naturally in certain fruits and veggies—including stone fruits, avocados, dried fruits, celery, and snap peas—and may be added to low-carb, keto, and/or sugar-free packaged foods like jams/jellies, candy/

confections, "no sugar added" frozen yogurt, low-carb/low-calorie ("healthy") ice creams, and low-carb protein bars.

The diarrhea that results from **malabsorption** of sugars and sugar alcohols is called **carbohydrate intolerance**, and refers to conditions like lactose intolerance, fructose intolerance, and sucrose intolerance—as well as to diarrhea and gas that result from excess intake of polyols. Its typical onset is four to eight hours after consuming a food with one of these sugars in it, with the severity of diarrhea contingent on the amount of sugar consumed. Consult Chapter 5 to learn more about osmotic diarrhea from these sugars; how to determine whether maldigestion of one or more of these sugars is contributing to your IBS-D symptoms; which foods contain which of these sugars; and what enzyme supplements might be available to help you better tolerate foods that contain certain of these sugars.

The Low-FODMAP Diet

The **low-FODMAP diet** is another common dietary approach for managing symptoms of IBS. FODMAP is an acronym for:

Fermentable *(a scientific way of saying that bacteria can break something down and make gas)*

Oligosaccharides *(refers to a variety of poorly digested carbohydrates found in certain grains, beans, and veggies)*

Disaccharides *(in this case, it refers to a sugar called lactose)*

Monosaccharides *(in this case, it refers to a sugar called fructose)*

And

Polyols *(also known as sugar alcohols, any sugar whose name ends with the suffix -ol)*

The premise behind a low-FODMAP diet is to reduce your intake of certain poorly absorbed carbohydrates—including fibers and some sugars—that gut bacteria can readily ferment, because when you feed the overgrowing bacteria, they'll produce lots of gas, bloating, and general digestive misery. Low-FODMAP fruits, vegetables, grains, proteins, and sugars are less fermentable by gut bacteria, so eliminating them can be a helpful way to manage bloating, abdominal pain, and diarrhea for many people with IBS.

The best available research suggests that 70% to 75% of people with IBS have a measurable degree of symptom improvement on the low-FODMAP diet, and more recent probing suggests that a scaled-down version of the low-FODMAP diet—sometimes referred to as a FODMAP gentle diet—can deliver the lion's share of benefits without requiring extensive, long-term restriction. The low-FODMAP diet is not intended to be followed in its strictest form indefinitely, but rather as a learning diet that allows people with IBS to pinpoint specific families of foods that seem to aggravate their symptoms more than others. I like to use it as a diagnostic tool to help my patients make informed decisions about which specific foods they may want to avoid to best manage their symptoms. As such, it has three phases: (1) a brief elimination phase, in which multiple families of poorly digested, fermentable carbohydrates are taken out of the diet for two to four weeks; (2) a re-challenge phase, in which you systematically reintroduce small portions of foods from a specific family of carbohydrates to determine whether these provoke symptoms; and (3) a maintenance phase, in which you incorporate tolerated higher FODMAP foods to your liking and continue to avoid only the ones that you've identified as a trigger. The diet and subsequent reintroduction process can be really hard to navigate alone; I strongly advise you to work with a registered dietitian trained on the low-FODMAP diet to make sure you have the support you need to go through the process and correctly identify your individual food triggers.

I've dedicated an entire chapter to the low-FODMAP diet in my first book, *The Bloated Belly Whisperer*, if you'd like a more detailed reference. Table 4-1 contains a very brief summary of which foods are highest in FODMAPs and therefore most likely to trigger symptoms in people with IBS.

Table 4-1: The Low-FODMAP Diet for Managing Symptoms of IBS-D

	High FODMAP (Limit/Avoid)	Low FODMAP (Allowed)
Fruits (and Juices Made from Them)	Apples	Bananas
	Apricots	Blueberries
	Blackberries	Cantaloupe
	Cherries	Clementines
	Dried fruits: apricots, dates, dried mango, figs, goji berries, prunes	Cranberries
		Coconut
		Grapes
	Figs	Guavas
	Lychees	Honeydew
	Mangoes	Kiwis
	Nectarines	Lemons, limes
	Peaches	Oranges, tangerines
	Pears	Papayas
	Persimmons	Pineapples
	Quinces	Plantains
	Watermelon	Raspberries
		Strawberries
		Tropical fruits: breadfruit, dragon fruit, mangosteen, passion fruit, star fruit (carambola)

(continues)

Table 4-1 *(continued)*

	High FODMAP (Limit/Avoid)	Low FODMAP (Allowed)
Vegetables	Artichokes Asparagus Avocados (up to $1/8$ avocado per sitting is OK) Beets Bitter melon Brussels sprouts Butternut squash Cauliflower Celery Chayote Fennel bulb Garlic (including garlic powder) Jicama Kale Leeks Mushrooms Peas Red cabbage or savoy cabbage Shallots Snow peas, sugar snap peas Sunchoke or Jerusalem artichoke Sundried tomatoes	Arugula Bamboo shoots Bean sprouts Bell peppers Bok choy Broccoli florets (not stalks) Cabbage (green) Carrots Cassava Chives, green onions, scallions, scapes (green part only) Collard greens Corn Cucumber Eggplant Endive Ginger Green beans/haricots verts/string beans Hearts of palm (palmitos) Lettuce—all varieties Lotus root Okra Olives Onions (including onion powder) Oyster mushrooms Root veggies: (celeriac, parsnips, radish, rutabaga, turnips, white potato) Seaweed (nori) Spinach Summer squash (yellow squash, zucchini) Sweet potato (limit portion to ½ cup) Swiss chard Taro Tomatillo Tomatoes Water chestnuts Winter squash (acorn, delicata, kabocha, pumpkin, spaghetti) Yucca (limit portion to ½ cup)

Table 4-1 *(continued)*

	High FODMAP (Limit/Avoid)	Low FODMAP (Allowed)

Grains and Starches	Any product, including gluten-free baked goods, that contains: bean/chickpea/lentil flour, chicory root fiber, inulin, soy flour, soy protein concentrate, tiger nut flour
	
	Barley
	
	Pumpernickel bread
	
	Regular wheat-based products: bread, cereals, couscous, crackers, farina, flour tortillas, pasta, pita, rolls, wraps
	
	Rye
		Buckwheat/kasha
		Corn/corn tortillas/cornmeal/grits/masa harina/polenta
		Gluten-free products made with any of these entries listed without added high-FODMAP ingredients:
		  Oat bran, oatmeal, oats
		  Potato/potato starch
		  Quinoa
		  Rice (all varieties)
		  Sorghum flour
		  Sourdough wheat or spelt bread
		  Tapioca starch (cassava flour)

(continues)

Table 4-1 *(continued)*

	High FODMAP (Limit/Avoid)	Low FODMAP (Allowed)
Proteins	Beans: black, kidney, pinto, white, and products made from them (bean-based pastas, falafel, hummus, veggie burgers, etc.) Cashews Dal/split peas Pistachios Protein powders: soy protein concentrate, whey protein concentrate Soy milk	Almonds (10/serving) Beef Chia seeds Chicken Chickpeas (up to ¼ cup canned/rinsed) Edamame (boiled soybeans), ½ cup Eggs Firm tofu Fish Flax seeds (up to 2 tsp) Hazelnuts (10/serving) Hemp seeds/hearts Lamb Lentils (up to ¼ cup canned/rinsed) Macadamia nuts Peanuts Pecans Pepitas/pumpkin seeds Pine nuts Pork Protein powders: collagen protein, hemp protein, pea protein isolate, pumpkin seed protein, rice protein, soy protein isolate, whey protein isolate Sesame seeds Shellfish Sunflower seeds Turkey Tempeh Walnuts

Table 4-1 *(continued)*

	High FODMAP (Limit/Avoid)	Low FODMAP (Allowed)
Dairy Foods and Dairy Substitutes	Buttermilk Condensed milk Cottage cheese Dulce de leche Evaporated milk Kefir/Yogurt Milk Oat milk (<½ cup is OK) Paneer Ricotta cheese Soy milk Vegan dairy substitutes made from cashews	Almond milk American cheese Butter/ghee Coconut milk beverage (up to ¾ cup) Cream cheese (limit to 2 TBSP) Hard/aged cheeses: Asiago, cheddar, Colby, Comte, feta Havarti, Manchego, Parmesan, Swiss Hemp milk Lactose-free cottage cheese Lactose-free ice cream Lactose-free kefir/yogurt Lactose-free milk Mozzarella Nondairy yogurts made from almond milk or coconut milk Queso fresco Rice milk (up to ¾ cup)

(continues)

Table 4-1 (continued)

	High FODMAP (Limit/Avoid)	Low FODMAP (Allowed)
Sweeteners	Agave nectar Chicory root fiber Corn syrup solids Erythritol Fructose Fruit juice concentrates Golden syrup High-fructose corn syrup (HFCS) Honey Inulin Invert sugar Lactilol Lactose Mannitol Pancake syrup Sorbitol Truvia (contains erythritol) Xylitol Yacon syrup	Acesulfame potassium Allulose Aspartame Barley malt syrup Brown rice syrup Brown sugar Corn syrup Dextrose Glucose Maple syrup (100% natural) Molasses Monkfruit extract (luohan guo) Saccharin Stevia (Reb-A) Sucralose (Splenda) Sugar (cane sugar, evaporated cane juice, palm sugar, sucrose)
Fats and Oils	Cream cheese (up to 2 TBSP is OK) Sour cream (up to 2 TBSP is OK)	All other fats and oils are allowed, including butter (Use fats and oils in moderation; fried foods or very high-fat foods may trigger IBS symptoms)

While many people with IBS-D avoid all FODMAP families for a period of time, it's actually lactose, fructose, and sugar alcohols that are most likely to trigger diarrhea as compared with other high-FODMAP carbohydrates. Non-sugar forms of high-FODMAP carbohydrates, called fructans and oligosaccharides, are more implicated in gas, bloating, and abdominal pain symptoms than they are in diarrhea.

Food Sensitivity

But what about the remaining 25% to 30% of people with IBS who feel they do have food triggers for their symptoms but do not respond adequately to some version of the low-FODMAP diet? Anecdotally, many patients with IBS report reacting very badly to specific foods—even if these foods are low-FODMAP and even if traditional allergy testing has not turned up any evidence of a **food allergy**. For example, I have many patients who become very symptomatic after consuming any amount of dairy—even if it's lactose-free (and therefore low-FODMAP) and despite having tested negative for a dairy allergy. Until recently, science hasn't been able to offer satisfactory explanations about why this might happen, and these reactions are usually classified vaguely as food sensitivities. Unfortunately, there hasn't been any scientifically valid way to diagnose such food sensitivities (see sidebar) with objective lab testing.

FOOD SENSITIVITY TESTING

A variety of tests claiming to identify nonallergic food sensitivities are especially popular among the alternative medicine crowd (think chiropractors, naturopaths, functional/integrative doctors, and nutritionists). Most are blood tests that measure an antibody called IgG, though there are other proprietary blood tests, that employ other methods, such as ALCAT testing, MRT tests, or "nutritional genomic" tests. Even some stool microbiome test companies offer diet advice based on the DNA of bacteria comprising your poop.

These tests are not evidence-based ways to diagnose food sensitivity or intolerance, or to derive science-based recommendations for diet. In fact, the IgG antibody levels that many food sensitivity test marketers claim indicate an intolerance have been used for years in the allergy/immunology world as a marker for food TOLERANCE! These are memory antibodies that are likely to be elevated for foods you eat regularly and foods your immune system has tolerance to.

As of the time of this writing, the only scientifically validated tests currently available for nonallergic food intolerances include breath tests for sucrose, lactose, or fructose intolerance (read about these in Chapter 5). Biopsies of the small intestine can also be taken to identify enzyme deficiencies for lactose, sucrose, or maltose digestion that can result in intolerance. For now, to identify all other suspected intolerances, an elimination diet with re-challenges is necessary.

While currently available food sensitivity tests aren't likely to produce reliable guidance about what foods trigger your IBS symptoms, there is a hypothesis that some subjectively reported food intolerances in a subset of people with IBS could indeed be the result of an atypical form of food allergy whose reactions are localized in the gut. By atypical, I mean that these are allergic-type reactions that are not carried out by the same IgE antibodies and white blood cells (mast cells and basophils) that classical food allergies are but rather by white blood cells called **eosinophils**.

A paper that explored this hypothesis was published in the journal *Gastroenterology* in 2020; it detailed a research study involving about one hundred people with IBS who reported a clear connection between eating certain foods and worsening symptoms. In the study, five potentially allergenic foods—wheat, milk, egg, soy, and yeast—were applied directly to the small intestinal surface of participants via endoscopy, and images of the tissue were captured immediately before and immediately after the application using technology called confocal laser endomicroscopy (CLE). CLE is basically a high-resolution microscope that's attached to an endoscope, allowing doctors or researchers to observe changes in your digestive system's lining in real time as if they were observing cells under a microscope in a lab. After the images were captured, tissue samples were collected so that they could also be analyzed outside the body in a lab. In this particular study, about 70% of participants had an observed reaction during the CLE procedure, with wheat being the most likely food to trigger a reaction. Interestingly, the patients who had these reactions did not experience IBS symptoms right away but rather several hours later. It is worth noting that none of these participants had tested positive for a traditional food allergy prior to being enrolled in the study. I imagine that we will learn a lot more about **atypical food allergies** and **eosinophilic gastrointestinal disorders (EGIDs)** as IBS triggers in the years to come, but suffice it to say that this could certainly explain the curious experiences of certain patients I've seen over the years who have reported almost immediate abdominal pain and cramping with even low-FODMAP forms of wheat or dairy and even after allergies and celiac disease had been ruled out. I always believed the patients' experiences; I was just never able to explain why they were having these experiences . . . perhaps until now.

Finally, the role of foods and beverages that directly stimulate the colon should be considered in any discussion of IBS: namely, coffee and alcohol. Both regular and decaffeinated coffee contains a compound called chlorogenic acid, which has a colon-stimulating effect; it's why so many of us can experience a pretty sudden urge to defecate within a sip or two of our morning cup of Joe. But in the case of IBS, in which the brain overinterprets routine signals from the gut with a heightened sense of alarm, the typical colon-stimulating effect of a cup of coffee can escalate into a full-on attack of constant colon spasms that result in extreme bowel urgency, cramping, and nonstop trips to the toilet all morning long. Contrary to popular belief, it's not actually the caffeine in coffee that exerts this effect, and someone with IBS is far more likely to be triggered by a decaf coffee than they would be by a caffeinated tea or cola.

Alcohol is known to loosen stools the morning after consumption, and this is for two reasons. First, alcohol is a direct gastrointestinal irritant. And second, alcohol impairs the reabsorption of water in the colon. This is not specific to people with IBS. However, many people with IBS find that alcohol hits them harder the next morning than just causing a slightly looser bowel movement and can trigger significant diarrhea for the better part of the day. Nonabsorbable carbohydrates in some alcoholic drinks like beer, rum, or certain mixers may also compound the digestive impact of alcohol on your gut. Soluble fiber supplementation (see the next section and Chapter 12 for more on this) on evenings you plan to drink may help mitigate the severity of morning-after diarrhea, but moderation with alcohol intake is advisable as well.

Dietary Supplements for Managing IBS-D

A few well-chosen, inexpensive, and easily accessible dietary supplements can make a substantial difference in certain IBS-D symptoms.

Supplemental Soluble Fiber

People who routinely suffer from excessively frequent, loose, crampy, and incomplete bowel movements in the first few hours of the morning often respond very well to a simple soluble fiber supplement taken at night. Two to four grams of supplemental **soluble fiber** taken in the evening—either in pill or powder form—are often sufficient to help consolidate those multiple, poorly formed, incomplete stools into one or two soft (but formed), long, and complete bowel movements the following morning. It often scares my patients who are already prone to frequent, loose, or urgent bowel movements when I suggest they take MORE fiber, and this is especially so since most fiber supplements are marketed as a constipation remedy. But you'll have to trust me on this one; soluble fiber supplements are routinely described as "life changing," especially by my patients who struggle with excessive toileting in the morning. See Table 12-1 on page 240 for more details on recommended brands and doses of soluble fiber for IBS-D.

Peppermint Oil Capsules

For people who struggle with urgent, crampy, post-meal bowel movements, taking **enteric-coated peppermint oil** pills one to two hours before an anticipated trigger situation can help prevent the spasmy urgency provoked by a meal. Others who experience chronic, constant, dull, achy, lower-abdominal pain also often respond well to peppermint oil capsules. Peppermint oil is a natural antispasmodic that helps relax smooth muscles—such as those that comprise the gut walls—and it has been demonstrated to be effective in reducing abdominal pain and cramping in people with IBS. "Enteric coated" refers to an acid-resistant pill coating that ensures your pill doesn't dissolve prematurely in the stomach before it can be delivered to its target site: the intestines. An effective dose should contain at least 0.2 mL of peppermint oil. In the United States, such products are marketed under the brand names IBgard, Heather's Tummy Tamers, Pepogest, and Atrantil; generic options are also available, as is a kosher/vegan product marketed by a company called Deva. If you typically experience diarrhea or urgent bowel movements after lunch, try taking peppermint oil before breakfast or midmorning a few hours after breakfast. If dinner is your danger zone, try taking it in the late afternoon. Take it before bed to help manage morning symptoms. You can take a 0.2 mL dose of encapsulated peppermint oil up to three times daily if necessary and well tolerated. **Pregnant women should not take peppermint oil supplements without first consulting their physician**, and some people with severe acid reflux find that even well-encapsulated peppermint oil capsules can still aggravate their reflux symptoms.

L-Glutamine Supplements

People with post-infectious IBS (see sidebar on page 50) in particular may have another potentially efficacious dietary supplement option: **L-glutamine**. There is a small amount of data suggesting that a portion of people with IBS-PI can experience improvement when given high doses of a dietary supplement called L-glutamine, which is an isolated protein building block (amino acid) that human gut cells particularly like to use as an energy source. A 2019 randomized controlled trial involving about a hundred people with diarrhea-predominant IBS-PI and published in the journal *Gut* found that about 80% of people in the group given a 5 g dose of supplemental L-glutamine three times daily for eight weeks reported significant improvements in their symptoms—specifically related to frequency of bowel movements and improved stool form—compared with only about 5% of people who were given a placebo supplement. On one hand, this is an extremely limited amount of data to base recommendations on. On the other hand, L-glutamine is among one of the safest types of dietary supplements one could imagine, provided your kidneys are well functioning and you don't need to follow a protein restriction. The typical American diet probably contains somewhere between three and six grams of glutamine anyway, just from food alone. Based on this study, I'd venture to say that it's worth trying for up to two months, and if you don't see any improvement, there's no compelling reason to keep using it.

Probiotic Supplements

People with IBS often ask me whether they should take a **probiotic**—and if so, which one. The data are not particularly strong with regard to demonstrating a benefit of specific probiotics for chronic diarrhea related to IBS-D, and to be honest, probiotic supplements are not a central part of my dietitian tool kit for managing IBS symptoms. It often shocks people to hear this, and I hear a lot of "but *they* say that probiotics are essential to gut health" from my patients. (I always question who this "they" are anyway, and oftentimes I find it's people trying to sell you probiotics.) If by "they," however, we mean the American Gastroenterological Association (AGA), you may be interested to know that in guidelines they published in 2020 based on a review of close to eighty studies on probiotics and IBS, they concluded that there wasn't enough evidence to warrant recommending them. Part of the issue is there are loads of really small studies that investigate a single strain or specific combination of strains at varying doses that show promise, but they are countered by other studies that show no benefit. What's more is that there are almost no studies that successfully replicate positive results with the same products in larger groups to validate the earlier findings. To complicate matters, probiotics research in IBS patients often measures a variety of different outcomes using a variety of different measurement tools. It's just really hard to draw any conclusions or make any reliable comparisons from such a messy body of literature.

To be clear, I am in no way dismissing the possibility that certain strains or combos of probiotic strains *could* be beneficial for certain people with IBS. In fact, I know for a fact that many of my patients over the years have stumbled upon a particular probiotic product that they feel has made a substantial positive impact on their IBS symptoms. I love it when that happens for them, as countless of my IBS patients over the years have tried a slew of probiotics and reported feeling no different . . . or actually even feeling worse. As of the time of this writing, I still have no good evidence to guide me about which patient might benefit from which probiotic, so probiotics trials basically amount to throwing proverbial spaghetti against the wall to see what sticks. As such, I tend not to waste my patients' time and money on the search when there are clearer, more evidence-based options for symptom management available.

If you still feel you really want to give the probiotics a try, here's what I can tell you. First, more recent reviews of the scientific literature on IBS and probiotics suggest that, in general, multi-strain probiotic cocktails are more likely to have a benefit than single-strain products. Second, specific strains from the *Lactobacillus* and *Bifidobacterium* groupings are most common among the cocktails of probiotics that produced a symptom improvement in various research studies; on a supplement facts label, these strains may appear listed with a capitalized and italicized "*L.*" or "*B.*" followed by a lowercase italicized Latin word. Third, it's really tricky to find commercially available probiotic products that match the specific strains or combinations of strains that were tested in many of the research studies conducted in various countries across the world, so even if a research study shows promise, there's a low chance you'll be able to walk into a store and buy something identical to the probiotic it tested. For this reason, you may want to look for (1) multi-strain cocktails that (2) contain at least one or more species from the *Lactobacillus* or *Bifidobacterium* categories, with (3) at least one or more strains from the species most commonly included in studies that have shown some benefit. They include: *Lactobacillus acidophilus*, *Streptococcus thermophilus* (which is also found in all yogurt), *Bifidobacterium breve*, and *Bifidobacterium longum*. It's still a crapshoot but maybe a little bit less of one.

One of the reasons that probiotics are so alluring as an IBS treatment is that it's long been presumed that some sort of alteration within the gut microbiota has a lot to do with the condition. While there's good evidence to suggest that imbalances in the gut microbiota of people with IBS are probably pretty complex and cannot be pinned to any one specific organism in a way that would allow for a quick silver-bullet solution, it has nonetheless been observed that people with IBS do seem to have lower amounts of bifidobacteria in their stool samples compared with healthy controls. Importantly, we also know that harboring higher levels of bifidobacteria is associated with having lower levels of abdominal pain—in both people with IBS as well as those without it. Therefore, logic tempts us to just supplement probiotic pills packed with these underrepresented species to bolster our inner ranks and help address IBS symptoms.

Prebiotic Supplements

This string of logic leads us to the next category of supplements that have been explored as potential treatments for IBS symptoms: **prebiotics**. Prebiotics are specific types of fiber that share some key common characteristics: they are highly fermentable by gut bacteria, and they are preferentially fermented by specific types of gut bacteria—namely, various species in the bifidobacteria and lactobacilli groups. Interestingly, ingesting prebiotic fiber seems to increase the abundance of these desirable bacterial species in the gut MORE effectively than probiotic supplements containing these very bacteria themselves! It certainly makes sense to consider that nourishing the species and strains already native to your own individual gut's ecosystem would be a more reliable way to bolster their ranks than trying to introduce some random outside organisms into an already-established ecosystem.

Prebiotic fiber can be found naturally in foods and is also added to foods or marketed in supplement form. Examples include inulin (chicory root fiber), fructooligosaccharides (FOS), galactooligosaccharides (GOS), resistant starch, and beta-glucans. When bacteria ferment these prebiotic fibers, they produce those highly desirable, anti-inflammatory short-chain fatty acids.

So, in helping to increase the abundance of *Bifidobacterium* species in the gut, do prebiotic fiber supplements actually help people with IBS-D to manage their symptoms? It's complicated. First is the question of whether a prebiotic supplement itself will provoke IBS symptoms. Anything fermentable has the potential to create a significant amount of gas, and many people with IBS can be extremely sensitive to the presence of even modest amounts of bowel gas. After all, prebiotic fibers are counted among two of the five families of so-called FODMAPs, dietary carbohydrates that many people find can worsen their IBS symptoms of gas, bloating, and abdominal pain.

The most common prebiotic you are likely to encounter added to foods and supplements is **inulin**, sometimes labeled as chicory root fiber, agave inulin, Jerusalem artichoke flour, tigernut flour, or yacon syrup. Chemically, it's just a long chain of fructose molecules that human beings lack enzymes to break apart. Inulin is also found naturally in wheat, onions, and garlic, and may be largely responsible for why some people with IBS find these foods to cause them gastrointestinal distress—namely gas, bloating, and abdominal pain. It's been pretty well established that supplemental inulin increases levels of bifidobacteria in human guts, and it seems to do so at doses as modest as 5 g per day. But prebiotics have barely even been studied in people with IBS as a treatment option, and inulin in particular has mostly just been explored in people with constipation-predominant IBS (**IBS-C**) as a possible remedy to help them go *more*. One small study of thirty healthy volunteers *without* IBS found that even relatively low doses of agave-derived inulin (5 g) provoked bloating, flatulence, and rumbling, and the severity of these symptoms increased at a dose of 7.5 g. Participants also had more stools per day on the 7.5 g dose. These findings support what I see in my clinical practice regularly: Inulin can be a really difficult form of prebiotic fiber to tolerate if you have IBS, and probably not the best choice as far as fiber supplements or potential diarrheal remedies go. Interestingly, though, a very small study of nineteen people with IBS published in 2021 in the journal *Gut* found that co-ingesting a psyllium fiber supplement along with a hefty dose (20 g) of inulin reduced gas production significantly compared with ingesting the inulin alone. Having suffered through the gassy aftermath of an inulin overdose once after ordering a bowl of sunchoke soup during NYC Restaurant Week, for the life of me I cannot fathom how they recruited nineteen people with IBS who were willing to take 20 g of inulin all at once.

There are some non-inulin-based prebiotic products marketed to people with IBS, claiming to improve bowel regularity and/or reduce abdominal pain, mostly on the basis of small, company-commissioned clinical trials. One such example is a proprietary type of prebiotic called B-GOS (marketed under the brand name Bimuno). When tested in people with IBS-like digestive complaints (not necessarily diagnosed with IBS), B-GOS appeared to *reduce* their complaints of abdominal pain, bloating, and gas more than a placebo product given to another group of participants. It did not change their stool consistency or bowel habits. Other studies of this prebiotic in healthy older volunteers confirmed that it resulted in increased levels of beneficial bifidobacteria compared with the patient's usual baseline levels and also compared with a placebo product. In other words, if you are interested in using a prebiotic fiber supplement to address gas and bloating but have found inulin to be poorly tolerated, this alternative product may be a reasonable option to consider. There's no good evidence to suggest it will reduce diarrhea, though.

Another such IBS-targeted category of prebiotics is known as **human milk oligosaccharides (HMOs)**. HMOs are lab-made molecules that mimic prebiotics found in breast milk and that have been shown to foster the growth of bifidobacteria in infants. They were first developed for use in infant formulas to allow these products to resemble breast milk more closely and provide health benefits to formula-fed babies, but they've since found their way into gut health supplements—particularly products marketed to people with IBS. A 2020 study involving 245 participants with IBS who were treated with an HMO prebiotic product marketed under the brand name Holigos IBS Restore found that they had a significant reduction in the percentage of their stools with abnormal consistency and a significant improvement in the severity of their overall IBS symptoms within the twelve-week study period, including a 50% reduction in the number of days with pain during the study period. There was no control group that was given a placebo with which to compare these results, though.

To be sure, all these itsy-bitsy studies on prebiotics and IBS don't necessarily warrant a hearty endorsement to include prebiotic supplements in your daily regimen—at least not yet. But given their well-established beneficial effect on bifidobacteria levels and the promising nature of early research findings, there is good reason to be optimistic.

Medical Approaches for Managing IBS-D

At present, there is no cure for IBS, but there are numerous over-the-counter and prescription medication options that are effective at helping people manage symptoms of diarrhea, too-frequent loose stools, and urgent, crampy bowel movements.

Antispasmodics

One commonly prescribed category of medication is **antispasmodics**. These medicines interfere with nerve stimulation of gut motility and slow down the colon's motility (also known as **anticholinergics**). These include medications like Bentyl (dicyclomine) and Levsin or Levbid (hyoscyamine); Librax contains two medications, Librium and clidinium, the latter of which is an anticholinergic. Bentyl is a medication that people will often take on a daily, more regimented basis—typically thirty to sixty minutes before each meal. It can help reduce an intestinal overreaction to the stimulation of eating, and reduce the likelihood of urgency, cramping, or diarrhea immediately following a meal. While hyoscyamine can be dosed similarly, its particular benefit is that it can also be taken as needed when a diarrheal attack strikes: It works within minutes. The medication is slipped under your tongue, where it rapidly enters the bloodstream and has an almost immediate spasm-stopping effect on the colon. As such, this is a medication that many people use on an episodic basis rather than as part of a daily regimen, and in my experience, sometimes the knowledge that you have a rapid-acting, effective remedy for sudden-onset diarrhea can provide a peace of mind that itself has a virtuous effect on preventing attacks to begin with. Antispasmodics are not appropriate for all people, and they can carry some side effects; you should discuss these with your gastroenterologist.

Antidiarrheals

In addition to antispasmodics, there are other **antidiarrheal** medications that work by preventing excessive fluid and electrolyte secretions from the intestinal cells into the colon. Lomotil (atropine and diphenoxylate) is one such prescription medication; it combines an anticholinergic (colon slower) with an antidiarrheal medication that works by preventing excess secretion of fluids and electrolytes from the intestinal cells into the bowel. Imodium (loperamide) is an over-the-counter medication with a localized opioid effect in the gut so that its action is limited to slowing down intestinal peristalsis—the smooth-muscle contractions that propel stool forward. This allows time for excess water in the bowel to be reabsorbed back into the body—helping to form stools—and should reduce the frequency of defecation as well. While many people with IBS-D will use loperamide only occasionally—to shut down their bowels if they need to be traveling, performing, or otherwise engaged in an activity in which they simply cannot afford to have an attack of diarrhea—some people with more severe cases of IBS-D include these medications as part of their daily regimen. Tolerance of these meds varies a lot by person. Some people with milder cases of IBS can sometimes find loperamide to work *too* well; while it definitely prevents attacks, it also may not wear off for a while, eventually leading to uncomfortable churning, cramping, or lower-abdominal pressure in which you may want to move your bowels for relief but cannot. Figuring out the right dose is key! A prescription medication called Viberzi (eluxadoline) works in a similar way. Pepto-Bismol and Kaopectate are both US brand names for bismuth subsalicylate, an antidiarrheal ingredient that also has a mild bacteria-killing effect; this makes it helpful for traveler's diarrhea, too. As the name suggests, bismuth subsalicylate contains salicylic acid, the active ingredient in aspirin, which has an anti-inflammatory effect. Bismuth subsalicylate can turn your stools blackish, so don't be alarmed by that surprising side effect. People who are allergic to aspirin or sensitive to salicylates should not use this medication.

Antidepressants

Unlike many of the above medications that can be used on an as-needed basis, some patients are treated with daily antidepressant medications. When antidepressants are prescribed to manage IBS-D, it's not because your doctor thinks that your symptoms are caused by stress or are "all in your head." It's because the medications that affect the nerves in your brain also affect the nerves in your gut, and these control movement and sensation of the gut. **Tricyclic antidepressant** medications (TCAs) like Elavil (amitriptyline), Pamelor (nortriptyline), and Norpramin (desipramine) are commonly prescribed, but the dose used to treat IBS-D is typically much lower than that prescribed to manage depression—at these lower doses, they are acting directly on the gut, not necessarily on your mood. Other antidepressant drugs in the selective serotonin reuptake inhibitor (SSRI) family, like Paxil (paroxetine hydrochloride), are also used to treat IBS-D. Serotonin-norepinephrine reuptake inhibitors (SNRIs) may sometimes be used to manage IBS-D when the diarrhea is accompanied by significant pain; they act both on the gut's motility as well as the brain-gut communication axis in which there is a tendency toward over-sensation leading to pain.

Antibiotics

In more recent years, an **antibiotic** called Xifaxan (rifaximin) was approved as a treatment for cases of IBS-D that do not respond adequately to other medications. This antibiotic differs from others in that it is not absorbed into the body but rather stays put and acts locally in the gut; it is also one of the most common treatments for small intestinal bacterial overgrowth; see Chapter 6. Clinical trials suggest that about 46% of people with IBS-D experienced improvement in both abdominal pain and frequency of loose or watery stools following a two-week course of rifaximin, and the average duration of improvement was about ten weeks (though within this subgroup of people who responded to the medication, a lucky 36% of them had symptom relief for a full six months). But here's the rub: In the

United States, Xifaxan is extremely expensive—a two-week course can cost over $1,000 as of the time of this writing—and it can only be prescribed three times total for the treatment of IBS-D. So even if you get a few months of relief from a single course of the medication, it's not necessarily going to be a viable long-term solution.

Behavioral Therapy Approaches for Managing IBS-D

Many people with IBS recognize that stress and anxiety can heighten their IBS symptoms. This is NOT to imply that IBS is a psychological condition or "all in your head" but rather that the brain and the gut are in constant communication, and for people with IBS, the brain is often overresponding to normal stimuli within the intestines—whether that be distension from larger meals, gas, or stool; chemical irritants like spices or alcohol; or the hormonal effect produced by a higher-fat meal. Likewise, the gut can overrespond to stress and anxiety signals that originate in the brain, whether with alterations in motility patterns or via a heightened sense of pain.

GI Psychology

The emerging field of **GI psychology** ("GI psych"), also known as psychogastroenterology, involves various behavioral therapies intended to "leverage the brain's ability to bring under voluntary control those symptom processes that seem, initially, to be driven completely by the gut," according to health psychologist Laurie Keefer, PhD, and her colleagues in a 2018 paper they published in the journal *Gastroenterology*. In other words, GI psych has two primary aims: to harness the brain as a partner in managing digestive symptoms, and to provide you with behavioral and coping tools that enable you to change thought and behavior patterns that worsen your health-related quality of life. GI psych interventions may be especially helpful for people who have noticed a particularly strong connection between their IBS symptoms and levels of stress and anxiety. Many academic medical centers now include GI psychologists as members of their gastroenterology departments.

Cognitive Behavioral Therapy

Cognitive behavioral therapy (CBT) is one such treatment option, and it provides tools to people with IBS that help them cope with pain or anxiety about the potential of having an attack at an inopportune time—while traveling, at work, or at a public event where restroom access is limited. Sometimes these fears can land people in a vicious cycle in which the brain and gut get stuck in a really dysfunctional loop: The brain becomes anxious about having an attack, which then precipitates an actual attack—a self-fulfilling prophecy of sorts—which then fuels more anxiety. CBT can give you tools to rewrite the script, so to speak, and change the thought patterns that feed into this self-defeating cycle. It involves working with a trained therapist to understand how your thoughts about various situations may drive your emotions, and how both of these can then affect physical sensations like hyperawareness of digestive sensations, increased pain levels, or even provoking actual attacks of cramping or diarrhea. There is a sizable and growing amount of research that supports the efficacy of CBT; about 50% of people with IBS seem to experience about a 50% reduction in their IBS symptoms with CBT, and this improvement lasts for years following a brief period of treatment.

Hypnotherapy

Gut-directed hypnotherapy is another modality that some people with IBS may be good candidates for as well. This behavioral health treatment actually helps retrain the brain to properly interpret signals from the gut, and some studies have shown it to be equivalent to the low-FODMAP diet in terms of efficacy in managing IBS symptoms. If you are suggestible (not everyone is!) and able to achieve a deep state of relaxation, a trained therapist can help guide you through a series of visualizations and suggestions that enlist the help of your subconscious mind to control physiological body processes—including gut motility or pain perception. For those people who do not have easy access to a medical hypnotherapist locally, there are some apps that may make this type of treatment more accessible. An app called Nerva offers a six-week, self-guided hypnotherapy program. A newer app called Regulora offers a twelve-week self-administered gut-directed hypnotherapy program developed by GI psychologists at the University of North Carolina aimed at reducing abdominal pain among people with IBS.

Diaphragmatic Breathing

Along with the strong evidence in support of some of the positive psychology interventions like CBT and gut-directed hypnotherapy described above, there is one surprisingly effective technique you can try practicing at home, for free, anytime, to help induce the nervous system's relaxation response and counteract the stress response's impact on the gut. **Diaphragmatic breathing** is a technique in which you practice deep, slow "belly breathing" as opposed to the shallower chest breathing to which we typically default. You can practice it anytime you feel yourself to be in a heightened state of stress and want to try resetting your gut's stress response back to a neutral place.

There are some excellent videos online that demonstrate the technique of diaphragmatic breathing; my favorite is from Megan Riehl, PsyD, from the University of Michigan; you can search for it online. The basic gist of it involves sitting comfortably or lying down with your eyes closed and gently placing one hand on your chest and the other hand on your belly. Start inhaling slowly through your nose to a count of four, paying attention to the fact that only your bottom hand on the belly will be moving as the belly expands outward; the chest should be still. Hold your breath for a count of two before starting to exhale slowly through your mouth for a slow count of six. Keep your mouth nice and relaxed as you exhale; no need to blow air out forcefully. Keep repeating this for anywhere from five to fifteen minutes, focusing on the rise and fall of your belly as you take these deep, slow breaths.

*

If you don't respond adequately to any of the standard dietary, medical, or other treatments for IBS-D, it is worth considering whether you may have been misdiagnosed. There are many conditions that present very similarly to IBS that are less common and therefore not routinely screened for. It's not at all unusual for patients to present with a diagnosis of IBS but then fail to respond at all to ANY of the dietary remedies I recommend or to any medical treatments their doctor has prescribed. In such cases, I will often collaborate with their doctor to consider testing or treating for other conditions that walk like IBS-D, talk like IBS-D . . . but are not, in fact, IBS-D. These include bile acid malabsorption (Chapter 6), small intestinal bacterial overgrowth (SIBO; Chapter 6), histamine intolerance (Chapter 8), and osmotic diarrhea from carbohydrate malabsorption (Chapter 5). Case studies of some such patients of mine are described in Chapters 6 and 8. If this resonates with your experience, I'd suggest reading those chapters to see if anything in them feels familiar.

Sugar Runs

*Osmotic Diarrhea
and Carbohydrate Intolerances*

I REMEMBER LEARNING ABOUT OSMOSIS sometime in junior high school science class. The teacher set up an experiment with several beakers filled with equal amounts of distilled water and added different amounts of salt to each one so that some were more concentrated and others less. We then added equal-size chunks of peeled, sliced potato to each of the beakers and checked on them at various time intervals. We observed that the higher the saltwater concentration of the saltwater bath, the smaller the potato chunk shrunk down. The shrinkage represented water from inside the potato being drawn out of the individual potato cell walls, attracted by the high concentration of salt in the beaker water.

This experiment demonstrated the concept of osmosis, or how water with lower levels of dissolved molecules will move across a semi-porous membrane toward water with higher levels of dissolved particles until the concentration of dissolved particles is the same on both sides. As more water was drawn out of the potatoes bathing in super-concentrated saltwater solutions, the potato chunks shrunk further.

Well, osmosis can happen in your intestines, too. The cells that line your colon are a semi-porous membrane—water can flow in and out of them. This means that when the contents passing through the colon have super-concentrated amounts of small particles—like, say, sugar molecules that went undigested and unabsorbed farther upstream in the small intestine—water is drawn from the cells that line the colon into the colon itself via osmosis. This can result in a type of diarrhea called **osmotic diarrhea**.

Osmotic Diarrhea from Carbohydrate Malabsorption (also known as the "Sugar Runs")

While many forms of diarrhea have their origin in something gone awry in the colon, or large intestine, diarrhea from the "sugar runs" actually originates farther upstream in the small intestine. The small intestine is where almost everything we eat is chemically broken down into elemental components by a variety of digestive enzymes and absorbed into the body by cells that line our intestines. Among the many nutrients absorbed in our small intestine are different types of sugars—namely, sucrose, lactose, maltose, fructose, and glucose. Food sources of these sugars are listed later in this chapter.

Fructose is just a single molecule that can be absorbed directly into gut cells by dedicated transporters that line the small intestine. Sucrose, lactose, and maltose are simple sugars made up of two molecules joined together by a chemical bond that first needs to be broken apart with enzymes before the component parts can be absorbed; these enzymes are produced on the spot by the hairlike tips of cells that line our small intestine, an area sometimes referred to as the brush border of the small intestine; see Figure 5-1 for an illustration of this. The enzyme that breaks apart sucrose into its component parts—one glucose and one fructose molecule—is called sucrase-isomaltase. The enzyme that breaks apart lactose into its component parts—one glucose and one galactose molecule—is called lactase. The enzyme that breaks apart maltose into its component parts—two individual glucose molecules—is called maltase.

83

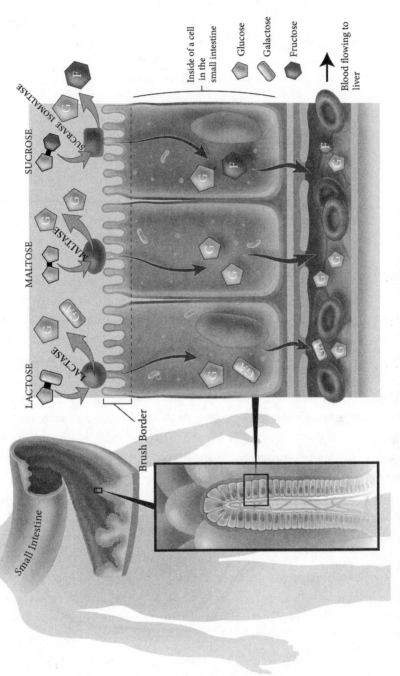

Figure 5-1: The sugar-digesting disaccharidase enzymes in the small intestine
Artwork by Mehtonen Medical Studios

(Some maltose is also broken down by the same sucrase-isomaltase enzyme that digests sucrose as well.)

A significant percentage of the US population may have trouble absorbing one or more of these sugars. Since sugars are a form of carbohydrate, we often refer to these conditions collectively as **carbohydrate malabsorption**. If you're counted among the group of people who malabsorb one of these carbohydrates and you happen to consume more of your problem sugar than your body is able to absorb in the small intestine, then these intact sugars will wind up in your colon. A high concentration of sugar in the colon will attract fluid from intestinal cells into the digestive tract through osmosis, and this results in the osmotic diarrhea described above.

Lactose intolerance is the best-known form of carbohydrate malabsorption, and many people suspect they're affected by it based on repeated instances of having diarrhea hours after consuming dairy-based foods high in lactose. Lactose-containing foods include regular milk, lattes, cappuccino, ice cream, certain whey-based protein powders, and desserts made with milk or condensed milk, like pudding, custard pies, or dulce de leche; see Table 13-1 on page 258 for a complete list. But other types of carbohydrate malabsorption are generally under-recognized. **Fructose intolerance** results from poor absorption of the sugar fructose, found in honey, agave nectar, processed foods and drinks containing high-fructose corn syrup, asparagus, and fruits like mango, figs, and cherries; see Table 13-2 on page 262 for a complete list. It affects an estimated 30% of Caucasians in the United States, to varying degrees. (Unfortunately, given long-standing racial biases in medical research, we don't have good estimates for prevalence of fructose intolerance among people of color.) **Sucrose intolerance** results from poor absorption of the sugar sucrose, which is found in cane/beet sugar, maple syrup, certain veggies (carrots, corn, onions, garlic, potatoes), and many fruits (bananas, apples, oranges, pineapple, guava); see Table 13-3 on page 268 for a complete list. Once thought to be a rare condition that is usually diagnosed in childhood, we are now realizing that a primary cause of sucrose intolerance, **congenital sucrose-isomaltase**

deficiency (CSID), is estimated to affect about 1% of the US population, but it affects up to 10% of people diagnosed with diarrhea-predominant irritable bowel syndrome (IBS-D). Less common, but also possible, would be **maltose intolerance**, which results from poor absorption of a sugar found in grain foods like wheat flour–based products (breads, crackers, cereals), spelt, cornmeal, barley, and rye, as well as beer, sweet potatoes, and molasses.

Another potential cause of osmotic diarrhea is overconsumption of carbohydrates called **sugar alcohols** (or **polyols**) that taste sweet like sugar but don't have the same structure as sugars; this means our body can't absorb them in the same way it can absorb other simple sugars like glucose or fructose. Examples include sorbitol, mannitol, maltitol, xylitol, erythritol, and lactitol. Certain sugar alcohols can be found naturally in fruits and vegetables, like sorbitol (avocados, apples, pears, and stone fruits) and mannitol (cauliflower, snow peas, and celery). Others, like erythritol, xylitol, and lactitol, are industrially produced from natural sources for the express purpose of sweetening processed foods and drinks—though sorbitol and mannitol are also manufactured in labs for use in food processing as well. See Table 13-4 on page 274 for a complete list of foods and drinks that contain sugar alcohols.

Sugar alcohols are very popular among marketers of low-calorie beverages, sugar-free/low-carb/keto desserts, and sugar-free gum and confections. Unlike real sugars, sugar alcohols can't be digested and absorbed by humans, so they practically have no calories. Because we can't absorb them, sugar alcohols won't raise blood sugar levels; this makes them an appealing choice for people with metabolic issues like prediabetes, type 2 diabetes, and polycystic ovary syndrome (PCOS). Sugar alcohols also don't promote tooth decay like real sugar does, which makes them an especially attractive sweetener for chewing gum. You can see why these are such appealing ingredients for food and beverage manufacturers to use.

If it seems like sugar alcohols are too good to be true, you'd be correct. There is a catch. Since human beings lack the ability to absorb sugar alcohols in our digestive tracts, they will arrive intact to the colon, and can exert a very strong osmotic effect there. In fact, sugar alcohols have long been used in medications to treat constipation due to their well-known laxative effect, and the naturally occurring sugar alcohols in prune juice are one of the reasons it's earned its reputation as a laxative aid!

How Do Symptoms of Osmotic Diarrhea from Carbohydrate Malabsorption Present?

The most common symptoms of carbohydrate malabsorption are gas (mostly farting), abdominal cramping, and loose stools or diarrhea, though nausea and vomiting are possible as well at very high intake levels. Symptoms do not occur immediately upon consuming a trigger food or drink, as the gas (from bacteria fermenting the unabsorbed sugar) and diarrhea (from osmosis caused by the unabsorbed sugar) doesn't set in until that unabsorbed sugar makes it all the way to your colon. This should take a minimum of two to three hours after consuming the offending food or drink, and more likely four to six hours if you consumed the trigger as part of a mixed meal. If you are a very habitual eater, then this time lag can be helpful in allowing you to pinpoint triggers. For example, a habitual eater who gets diarrhea almost every single day at around 2 p.m. might want to look four to six hours backward and note what they ate between 8 a.m. and 10 a.m. to narrow down the likeliest culprit. With carbohydrate malabsorption, your loose stools or diarrhea may have a lighter color than normal, too: light brown, tan, or even a bit orangey. You may notice that your stools feel acidic on the way out, or they may leave your delicate anal tissue feeling itchy or irritated.

Symptoms of lactose, fructose, sucrose, or maltose malabsorption are generally the same, and will be dose dependent. This means that if you consume a small portion of your trigger sugar, you may only experience mild symptoms. If the symptoms are mild enough and happen several hours after you consumed the trigger food, you may not even make the connection. But as the portion you consume gets larger, the symptoms will become more severe. Similarly, the symptoms can be cumulative. This means that if you are, say, sucrose intolerant, and consume a high-sucrose food like pancakes with maple syrup at breakfast and then maybe have a mid-morning snack of a large banana, the diarrhea will be significantly worse later in the day than if you had eaten only one of these foods alone. Severe osmotic diarrhea from a high dose of malabsorbed sugar can be strong enough to wake you overnight or result in fecal incontinence (an accident) if you can't make it to a bathroom in time. Unlike the malabsorptive conditions described in Chapter 6, however, carbohydrate malabsorption may not cause much, if any, unintended weight loss.

One clue that you might be dealing with sucrose malabsorption in particular would be if you had attempted to follow a low-FODMAP diet for IBS (see page 57) and wound up feeling *worse*, not better. This is because the primary sugar you're allowed to consume on a low-FODMAP diet is sucrose, so by eliminating most other forms of sugar, you could wind up consuming more sucrose than usual and feeling all the worse for it. Similarly, a clue that you could be dealing with a sugar alcohol intolerance would be if you experienced an uptick in diarrhea after attempting to follow a keto or other very-low-carb diet that had you swapping out your usual snacks or treats with multiple sugar-free options sweetened with sugar alcohols. Since many of these products contain significant amounts of sugar alcohols, consuming several servings per day could give anyone quite a case of diarrhea!

Your age at the time of symptom onset is also worth mentioning as a potential clue to the presence of carbohydrate malabsorption. Sucrose intolerance is generally a genetically determined condition you are born with, which means you may have a lifelong history of being gas or diarrhea prone. The onset of lactose malabsorption typically appears at some point between late childhood or adolescence and into your twenties if you are genetically predisposed to wind down your lactase-making capacity with age, as the majority of humans on this planet are. It can also occur post-pregnancy and following a bout of viral gastroenteritis—what we commonly call stomach flu. If you make it to age thirty without having developed symptoms of lactose intolerance, you're probably home-free; it would be pretty unusual to develop lactose intolerance in midlife or beyond unless it was secondary to (caused by) another medical condition. In fact, if you do start to notice that you're becoming diarrhea prone following dairy consumption later in adulthood, it may not be a bad idea to get checked out for giardiasis (infection with a parasite called *Giardia*), celiac disease, or small intestinal bacterial overgrowth (both Chapter 6) to make sure that your new lactose intolerance isn't actually a reversible side effect of something else.

Diagnosing Osmotic Diarrhea from Carbohydrate Malabsorption

Breath Testing

The most common way to diagnose lactose, fructose, and sucrose intolerance is a noninvasive, safe method called **breath testing**. These tests can be conducted in a doctor's office—and are increasingly available for self-administration at home. A properly conducted lactose or fructose intolerance test should last for three hours and should be conducted following an overnight fast. After breathing into a bag to capture a baseline sample of your breath gases when fasted, you will then drink a solution with 25 grams of either lactose or fructose. Then, every fifteen to thirty minutes for the next three hours, you will breathe into a bag, and the gases you've exhaled will be fed into a machine that can quantify the amount of hydrogen (H_2) and methane gas (CH_4) contained within. Hydrogen and methane gases are not produced by human cells, so if they're in your breath, we know that bacteria produced them in response to something you fed them. If you did not absorb the lactose or fructose consumed at the beginning of the test, then once these sugars arrive to the colon—usually at some point between hours two to three of the test—we would see a spike in the amount of one or both of these gases in your breath samples that's indicative of bacterial fermentation. If you are found to be a lactose or fructose malabsorber based on this test, you should expect to experience some pretty unpleasant gas and diarrhea toward the end of the test or very soon after it's completed. Don't say you weren't warned.

I've seen a fair number of shenanigans when it comes to lactose and fructose breath testing, so it's worth mentioning them here. First, tests shorter than three hours cannot accurately diagnose lactose or fructose malabsorption. Second, drinking a can of Coca-Cola or a glass of milk at home and then coming to a doctor's office a few hours later to provide breath samples is not an accurate way to diagnose fructose or lactose malabsorption, since it does not capture a baseline reading of the gases on your breath prior to starting the test. Finally, if you happen to have a condition called SIBO (Chapter 6), then you may have a false-positive breath test result for lactose or fructose malabsorption. One way to tell that this may be the case is if the numbers in your lactose or fructose breath test shoot up within the first ninety minutes of the test. Gases that appear this early in a breath test are being generated in your small intestine, not in your colon, and may signal that you're harboring an excess of bacteria there. Another tip-off is if you are tested for both lactose and fructose malabsorption and *both* tests come back strongly positive, especially if they go positive within the first ninety minutes.

While some clinical practices offer a similar hydrogen breath test to diagnose sucrose malabsorption (it uses 50 g of sucrose and follows the same protocol as described above for lactose and fructose intolerance), a different type of test called the ^{13}**C-sucrose breath test (SBT)** may be more accurate. This test involves drinking a solution that contains a special form of sucrose that has been labeled with a unique form of carbon called ^{13}C. If you consume this special form of labeled sucrose (^{13}C-sucrose), then we'd expect to see a specific amount of specially labeled carbon dioxide ($^{13}CO_2$) on your exhaled breath after your body finishes breaking it down and metabolizing it. If you do not absorb the test sucrose completely, then a lower-than-expected amount of the labeled carbon dioxide will appear on your breath. As this explanation suggests, the ^{13}C-sucrose breath test requires you to drink a sugar solution and breathe into a certain number of test tubes over a ninety-minute period. The breath samples will be analyzed by a lab, and can determine whether your enzyme activity level is normal or not based on the type of carbon dioxide gas observed.

Small Bowel Biopsies

Lactose, sucrose, and maltose intolerance can also be diagnosed by having biopsies (tissue samples) of your small intestine taken during an upper **endoscopy** procedure, in which a gastroenterologist inserts a thin, flexible scope down your esophagus, through your stomach, and into your small intestine. Your gastroenterologist will take a few biopsies of the region of your small intestine where the digestive enzymes lactase, sucrase-isomaltase, and maltase are produced. These samples are sent to a lab where the level of enzymes present can be measured. If enzyme levels are lower than normal, it can help diagnose malabsorption of one or more of these sugars. This test is called a **disaccharidase assay**.

Treating Osmotic Diarrhea from Carbohydrate Malabsorption

There's no real way to stop osmotic diarrhea once it has started; you just have to wait it out until your body has passed the undigested load of whatever sugars or sugar alcohols you consumed. For this reason, prevention is the only management strategy.

Dietary Treatments for Osmotic Diarrhea from Carbohydrate Malabsorption

Once you've figured out which sugars trigger your diarrhea, you'll need to avoid them to the greatest degree possible. There are enzyme supplements for certain sugars that may aid in their digestion and absorption. If such an option is available for your trigger sugar(s), then you may not need to avoid foods that contain it/them entirely, so long as you take an appropriate dose of an appropriate enzyme with your food. See the section on supplements and medical treatments for more details on using enzymes properly to manage carbohydrate intolerances.

Chapter 13 contains detailed tables of which foods contain which sugars so that you can identify a list of safe foods to consume freely based on your individual sugar triggers, and know which foods that either need to be avoided or paired with an appropriately matched enzyme product. When you finish reading this chapter, flip ahead to Chapter 13 to see the food lists, sorted by type of sugar.

No human being can absorb sugar alcohols, and there are as yet no dietary enzymes that make them absorbable. In other words, any of us who consumes a large-enough portion of sugar alcohols will eventually develop diarrhea; if you don't believe me, google product reviews for sugar-free gummy bears and you will see for yourself. Some people are much more sensitive to them than others, though. If you are very diarrhea prone, it's a good policy to avoid foods and sweetened beverages that have added sugar alcohols (see Table 13-4 on page 274). You might consider keeping your portions of fruits and veggies that naturally contain sugar alcohols somewhat conservative as well.

Dietary Supplements for Osmotic Diarrhea from Carbohydrate Malabsorption

Over-the-counter supplements called **digestive enzymes** can be helpful in improving tolerance to your problem food if you take them within a few minutes of starting to consume a food that contains your trigger. Digestive enzymes are specific to their targets. In other words, an **enzyme** only works if it's the right enzyme for the job you need it to do. For this reason, randomly chosen digestive enzyme blends may or may not be useful to you in trying to manage a specific carbohydrate intolerance. The devil is in the details:

You need to choose a product that contains an effective dose of the enzyme tailored to digest your problem sugar in order for it to work. If you have been able to isolate a very specific sugar that gives you trouble through breath testing or small bowel biopsy, you may be better off using a product that contains ONLY the enzyme ingredient you need, as the dose of the effective ingredient will almost certainly be higher. For example, if you are lactose intolerant, you can easily find lactase enzyme products that contain 6,000 to 9,000 units of lactase per pill. If you were to buy a digestive enzyme cocktail that contained a dozen different enzymes in it, there may be less than 1,000 units of lactase per pill to make room for lots of other enzymes you don't even need. This lower dose may not be enough to cover the portion of food you're consuming.

Lactase enzyme: Research suggests that a dose of at least 3,000 ALU (acid lactase units) should cover a reasonable portion of lactose-containing dairy, but 6,000 to 9,000 ALU would be even better. Some brands use sugar alcohols like mannitol as inactive ingredients in their lactase enzyme supplements; if you are diarrhea prone, I'd advise you to choose a brand without fillers that end in the letters *ol*.

Glucose isomerase (or **xylose isomerase**) is an enzyme that converts fructose to more absorbable glucose, and can help manage symptoms of fructose intolerance. The small amount of available research suggests that a dose of 130 mg of this enzyme was sufficient to cover a dose of 25 g of fructose in a small group of study participants with fructose intolerance. This is roughly the amount in a typical can of soda. A European product marketed under the brand name Fructaid (Pro Natura) is available for purchase online in the United States; it contains 50 mg of enzyme per pill, so you may need to experiment with effective dosing for your preferred foods.

Some newer enzyme cocktails are available that contain both lactase and glucose isomerase in a single pill, along with other enzymes. These can be incredibly convenient if you experience both lactose and fructose intolerance, provided that the doses they contain are adequate to cover your typical intake. One such example is FODMATE enzyme (Microbiome Labs). Each two-pill dose contains 10,000 ALU of lactase and an undisclosed dose of glucose isomerase to digest fructose. It also contains bonus enzymes that help digest typically gassy carbohydrates found in foods like onions, garlic, wheat, beans, and brussels sprouts and may be helpful for people with IBS who have found that a low-FODMAP diet (see Chapter 4) helps manage their symptoms of gas, bloating, and/ or diarrhea but for whom long-term adherence to this diet is not possible. A similar product called FODZYME (Kiwi Biosciences) contains a similar cocktail of FODMAP-digesting enzymes, but without the fructose-digesting one. As of the time of this writing in late 2022, there are no supplemental enzyme products available that render sugar alcohols (polyols) digestible. However, according to their website, Kiwi Biosciences is developing such a novel ingredient to add to their FODZYME product. If they succeed, it would be the first of its kind! Until then, if sugar alcohols give you grief, you'll do well to steer clear of foods that contain them; see Table 13-4 on page 274 for a list.

It is unclear whether available over-the-counter enzyme supplement products are effective at managing sucrose intolerance. Some enzyme cocktails contain an ingredient called invertase, which is a yeast-derived enzyme that breaks sucrose apart into its component parts; it's used sometimes in food processing. Unlike dietary supplements that contain lactase and glucose isomerase, however, dietary supplements of invertase seem not to have actually been tested in people with known sucrose intolerance to see if this enzyme is effective within the human body to manage symptoms of sucrose intolerance. A prescription option is available; it is described in the following section.

Medical Treatments for Osmotic Diarrhea from Carbohydrate Malabsorption

There is a prescription enzyme product called Sucraid (sacrosidase) available for people with sucrose intolerance due to sucrase-isomaltase deficiency. It comes in liquid form with a dropper and is to be diluted in a small amount of water and consumed immediately before a sucrose-containing meal. Still, my patients with sucrose intolerance often need to employ a hybrid strategy of using their Sucraid when it is convenient, and knowing how to avoid high-sucrose foods and drinks when traveling or when it's not feasible to carry their enzymes with them.

Case Study: Melanie's Carbohydrate Intolerances Masked by Constipation

Melanie was a woman in her late twenties referred to me by her gastroenterologist for help solving a yearslong digestive mystery: What was causing her out-of-the-blue attacks of extremely urgent, watery diarrhea that struck only once every four to six weeks? The weird thing about these diarrhea attacks was that as soon as the diarrhea was out of her, she felt totally fine. Her gastroenterologist had already ruled out the more serious stuff—celiac disease and inflammatory bowel disease—before sending her my way for a dietary evaluation.

The diarrheal attacks seemed totally bizarre to Melanie, especially since she'd actually been constipation prone her entire life. As a kid, she used to run so constipated that her pediatrician put her on daily doses of MiraLAX. After that, she'd been able to move her bowels daily, though the MiraLAX did make her normal stool quite soft. These softer stools were never urgent, not "diarrhea," and she felt a good sense of relief when she finished going. Because of her baseline tendencies toward constipation and episodes of random diarrhea, she carried a diagnosis of IBS-M—or mixed type IBS.

First and foremost, I took a detailed history of Melanie's usual diet and asked her to recall which foods she remembered eating when the last several diarrhea attacks occurred. Her daily diet was pretty varied, though I noted she ate quite a bit of dairy. I wondered whether lactose intolerance could be contributory to her diarrhea, though it seemed likely that if it were, she'd be having diarrhea way more often than once every four to six weeks. When I examined foods associated with specific attacks of diarrhea, there did seem to be a common thread around many of the meals being high-histamine ones—aged cheese, tomato sauce, spinach, and wine—and this made me think of histamine intolerance as a possible trigger (Chapter 8). However, her usual daily diet also included plenty of high-histamine foods in it, and she wasn't having diarrhea daily or even weekly, so that hypothesis seemed less likely.

To start, I figured we should make sure we weren't dealing with overflow or dam-breaking diarrhea (described in Chapter 3) related to Melanie being unknowingly backed up, so I asked her gastroenterologist if he'd be open to ordering an X-ray that would show us whether she was full of stool. It turns out, she wasn't at all. Once I knew she wasn't backed up, I tried her on a fiber supplement to help firm up the stool. It made her feel gassy and bloated and had no effect on stool form or diarrheal episodes. (Sorry, Melanie.)

Next, I figured we should rule out malabsorptive conditions that might be set off by particularly large, higher-fat meals like many of the ones that seemed to be underway when her diarrhea struck—namely pancreatic insufficiency and small intestinal bacterial overgrowth (SIBO), both detailed in Chapter 6. Her doctor tested her for both, and they came back negative. While all these tests were underway, I suggested Melanie eliminate lactose-containing dairy for two to four weeks to see if anything changed. She reported that she was about 50% less gassy and bloated than her usual baseline, but there was no change in bowel patterns or stool consistency.

As I was mulling over my next move, Melanie and I got to talking about her sweet tooth, and she mentioned that she loved candy, but noticed that eating more than about two to three gummy worms always gave her diarrhea several hours later. This information had NOT come up in our initial daily diet recall, and it was just the piece of missing information I needed. I suggested that her doctor test her for sucrose intolerance and/or lactose intolerance to see whether malabsorbing these simple sugars was creating osmotic diarrhea that overpowered her constipated tendencies.

Melanie's doctor decided to conduct an endoscopy so he could obtain biopsies of her small intestine and measure the levels of all the sugar-digesting enzymes that are manufactured there: lactase, sucrase-isomaltase, and maltase. It was well worth the effort: it turns out Melanie was profoundly deficient in both lactase and sucrase-isomaltase enzymes, making her both lactose and sucrose intolerant.

With this new diagnostic information, we emerged with a clearer understanding of Melanie's diarrhea. Since she was malabsorbing both lactose AND sucrose (table sugar), on days she consumed larger amounts of one or both of these two sugars earlier in the day—cumulatively at breakfast and lunch and/or with snacks—she was likely provoking a diarrhea attack that would hit around dinnertime, right as the early day's undigested nutrients were arriving to her colon. What she happened to be eating at the time of the attack was completely irrelevant.

One of the lessons I drew out from this really tricky case, which took several tries to figure out, is how challenging it can be to identify malabsorbed sugars as a diarrhea trigger when someone's diet differs a lot from day to day—especially since the symptoms of sugar malabsorption tend not to occur for many hours after the trigger food was consumed. In Melanie's case, it seemed that low-grade daily symptoms of carbohydrate intolerance (gassiness and mushier stools) were being attributed to her tendency toward constipation and use of MiraLAX. It was only when Melanie had a massive diarrheal attack that we knew to look for carbohydrate intolerances as an underlying cause.

6

Malabsorptive Mayhem

Bile Acid Diarrhea, SIBO,
Celiac Disease, and Pancreatic Insufficiency

THERE ARE MANY CIRCUMSTANCES IN which something that is
supposed to be absorbed in the small intestine isn't. These episodes
of malabsorption can wreak a whole lot of havoc farther downstream
in the colon, resulting in diarrhea and strangely textured (sticky,
tarry, an absolute mess to wipe) or light-colored stools that may
float. Depending on the nature of the malabsorption, you may
also experience weight loss, nutritional deficiencies, large amounts
of intestinal gas (farting) with bloating or gas pain, and even fecal
incontinence (pooping accidents). Diarrhea from malabsorptive
causes often does not respond adequately to the usual diarrhea
remedies—like antidiarrheal medications or diet change—but will
generally let up if/when you are completely fasted for a day. If
you're not eating or drinking, after all, there's nothing to malabsorb!
Malabsorptive diarrhea from any of the causes described in this
chapter can also wake you overnight, and this is one key factor that
differentiates it from irritable bowel syndrome (IBS).

The four conditions described in this chapter that cause malabsorptive diarrhea have very different causes and very different
treatments. So why did I choose to lump them together in a single

chapter? It's because the way they present symptom-wise can have lots of overlap, and it can be hard to differentiate what is causing these symptoms without further testing. Your quiz results sent you to this chapter due to a cluster of symptoms that appear consistent with malabsorption of some type, but you will need to read about all the conditions to see which one(s) seem to resonate most with your experience. I'd also add that these four conditions are not mutually exclusive! It is common for people with celiac disease or pancreatic insufficiency, both described later in this chapter, to develop SIBO before they are diagnosed and properly treated. Similarly, bile acid malabsorption can occur independently or as the result of SIBO. When there are signs of malabsorption, your doctor may need to do a more comprehensive assessment that involves stool testing, blood testing, breath testing, and/or endoscopy to get a clear picture about what's causing it.

Bile Acid Malabsorption (BAM) and Bile Acid Diarrhea (BAD)

Bile acids are an ingredient in a digestive fluid called bile, which is produced by our liver to assist with fat digestion. Bile acids help emulsify large fat droplets into smaller fat droplets, so that more of their surface area can be exposed to fat-digesting enzymes during the digestive process in the small intestine. This enables more efficient fat absorption.

Bile is secreted by the liver. It travels to the small intestine through the common bile duct. It can be stored in the gallbladder (if you have one), and its release is stimulated by starting to eat. Once bile has done its digestive job, it's broken down into its component parts, and the bile acids it contains are supposed to be absorbed back into the body in the tail end of the final section of the small intestine—a segment called the terminal ileum. The bile acids that are reabsorbed travel right back to the liver so it can make new bile from them. Recycling at its finest!

But there are several circumstances in which these bile acids are not adequately reabsorbed into the body in the small intestine, which means they remain in the digestive tract and keep traveling onward into the colon. This is called **bile acid malabsorption (BAM)**. Perhaps your terminal ileum is inflamed from a case of Crohn's disease (see Chapter 7); as it happens, an inflamed terminal ileum is lousy at recycling bile acids. Certain medications can cause bile acids to be malabsorbed, including a commonly prescribed drug for pre-diabetes, type 2 diabetes, and polycystic ovary syndrome (PCOS) called metformin. Overgrowth of bacteria in your small intestine (see SIBO in the next section of this chapter) can also make bile acids more difficult to absorb, leading to bile acid malabsorption. Perhaps you've had a previous intestinal surgery in which the terminal ileum was cut out entirely so that there's no place for the bile acids to be reabsorbed. Or maybe you've had your gallbladder removed surgically, and your liver has since decided to overcompensate for its loss by providing a constant, steady drip of bile directly into your intestines at all times, thereby overwhelming your body's limited re-absorptive capacity. (Available data suggest that bile acid diarrhea affects up to 6% of people following gallbladder removal surgery; older studies have suggested an even higher percentage.) Then, there's the possibility that you just lost the genetic bile acid recycling lottery, and you were born with a small intestine that doesn't do a very good job at this task.

When bile acids find their way into the colon, they stimulate the colon's cells to secrete fluids and prompt increased motility of the colon. The result is mushy, frequent stools—or overt diarrhea. This is called bile acid diarrhea (BAD), and it is estimated that up to 25% of people who have been diagnosed with diarrhea-predominant **irritable bowel syndrome (IBS-D)** may actually be experiencing this condition instead! In this manner, bile acid malabsorption can be considered an IBS-mimicker . . . but is not actually IBS.

How Does Diarrhea from Bile Acid Malabsorption Present?

Urgency is the primary symptom associated with bile acid malabsorption (BAM), whether or not the stools themselves are actually diarrheal. In some cases, your stools can have some form to them, but remain way too frequent and way too urgent. People with BAM often report occasional episodes of fecal incontinence—or such urgency that they don't make it to the bathroom in time. Diarrhea from BAM is called bile acid diarrhea, or **cholerrhea**.

If stools have some form to them, they may be a sticky or messy texture; some people describe them as resembling soft-serve ice cream or cow patties. They can be hard to wipe clean. With bile acid malabsorption, diet change doesn't typically make much of a difference; neither do fiber supplements or IBS medications. While diet change can't typically make diarrhea from BAM go away entirely, certain diets can certainly make it worse. Specifically, high-fat foods or keto-style high-fat/low-carb dietary patterns can make it much worse. Abdominal pain seems to affect about half of people with BAM as well.

If your stools changed following surgery to remove your gallbladder or since starting (or increasing your usual dose of) a medication called metformin, you should suspect bile acid malabsorption as a possible culprit.

Diagnosing Bile Acid Malabsorption (BAM)

Experts tend to agree that BAM is underdiagnosed, and one of the likely reasons for this is that we haven't had a widely available diagnostic test for it here in the United States. In Europe, a test called ^{75}Se-Homocholic acid taurine (^{75}SeHCAT) scintigraphy has been available to diagnose the condition—but this is not currently an option for those of us on this side of the proverbial "Pond." (The test is quite time-consuming and costly, as it involves two visits to a radiologist one week apart after swallowing a capsule that contains a radioactive tracer.) As you might imagine, things that can't be easily tested for are often less likely to be considered early on in the diagnostic process. As such, a diagnosis of BAM often arrives after loads of other tests come back normal, and after the diarrhea fails to respond to any standard antidiarrheal medication, IBS treatment, or diet change attempted. Traditionally, in clinical practice here in the United States, a diagnosis of BAM would be confirmed by a positive response to the medication used to treat it: bile acid sequestrants. This may be changing, however. A stool test has recently been validated for diagnosing bile acid malabsorption. It is called the 48-hour fecal bile acid excretion test and involves following a high-fat diet for several days, during which time you collect all the stool you pass for forty-eight hours, to be analyzed in a lab.

Treating Bile Acid Diarrhea

Bile acid diarrhea doesn't really respond adequately to diet change, though certainly you can make symptoms a lot worse by consuming very high-fat foods. Bile acid diarrhea provoked by an especially high-fat meal will usually present many hours later—which is why some people can experience overnight diarrhea or severe morning symptoms following a richer dinner. Still, since bile is released all day long in response to eating, many people with BAD experience urgent, loose, sticky, or diarrheal stools multiple times throughout the day.

The only real treatment for BAD is to take a type of medication called a bile acid sequestrant, which binds to those irritating bile acids in the intestine and prevents them from stimulating fluid release and excessive motility in the colon. Common brands of bile acid sequestrants include a powder called Questran (cholestyramine) or pills called Colestid (colestipol) and Welchol (colesevelam). Of course, if the BAD is a side effect of medication use (like metformin) or SIBO, the condition will resolve when the underlying cause is corrected. You'll know within just a few days of using a bile acid sequestrant whether your diagnosis is confirmed, though often it can take some experimentation with dosing and timing of your medication to optimize symptom control. Too high a dose of the medication can be constipating, too low a dose will predispose you to breakthrough symptoms. Many of my patients will take a small dose two to three times daily rather than a single large dose in the morning to help ensure all-day coverage. I often encourage patients to consider adding an extra little top-off dose before meals that are especially large or high in fat—like those at parties, holiday or birthday celebrations, or just any particularly rich meal.

Case Study: Corinne's IBS Misdiagnosis

Corinne was a woman in her fifties who came to me with a lifelong history of "IBS" that she never really figured out how to manage. Her main symptom was extremely urgent diarrhea, and she would often skip meals to avoid triggering it when she knew she would not be near a toilet. Over the years, Corinne developed a hunch that fiber might have made her diarrhea worse—especially salads— so she tended to regard sandwiches and bread as her safe foods. Still, even when sticking to these foods, Corinne remained symptomatic in unpredictable ways. Over the years, she'd tried every elimination diet, numerous IBS medications, antidiarrheals, fiber supplements. Nothing ever really helped much.

Because Corinne had been avoiding most fruits and vegetables for the better part of her life, she felt it was difficult to manage her weight. More frustrating still, a prior attempt to follow a keto diet for weight loss provoked her diarrhea in the absolute worst possible way.

As soon as I heard Corinne's retelling of her lack of response to IBS treatments and her awful reaction to a high-fat keto diet, I wondered whether she even ever had IBS to begin with. It sounded to me like Corinne might actually have had bile acid diarrhea. When I shared this thought with her, a light bulb went off. Apparently, she had just recently met with a new gastroenterologist who had raised the same possibility. With both of her new providers now suggesting bile acid diarrhea as a possibility, Corinne was on board to trial a bile acid sequestrant medication called cholestyramine.

The results were almost immediate, though it took us a few weeks to play around with the optimal timing and dosing of the medication. Corinne's bowel movements normalized within days of starting cholestyramine, and there was no more urgency. The hardest part for Corinne was actually adjusting her mindset around safe foods; she remained terrified to eat a salad or very much fruit after decades of assuming they were diarrhea triggers. It took many months for Corinne to build her confidence that the medication would keep her regular no matter how much fiber she ate, and it remains an ongoing process to unlearn a lifetime of eating habits and relearn a new set of habits for the decades ahead.

For me, the big lesson from Corinne's story is that when someone is told they have IBS but they don't respond to a single dietary or medication intervention commonly used to manage IBS, one has to wonder whether the diagnosis is actually correct. Bile acid malabsorption is a surprisingly common IBS mimicker.

Small Intestinal Bacterial Overgrowth (SIBO)

In my first book, *The Bloated Belly Whisperer*, I dedicated an entire chapter to SIBO, but we've got a lot of ground to cover in this book, so I'll try to be more succinct here. As you'll recall from the diagram of your intestines in Chapter 2, a healthy, normal small intestine is supposed to harbor significantly fewer bacteria than the colon—and the more upstream regions of the small intestine (the duodenum and jejunum) are supposed to have even fewer bacteria than its downstream regions (the ileum). In fact, our bodies have many guardrails in place to help ensure that bacteria can't overpopulate our small intestine—from stomach acid and pancreatic fluids that have a natural antimicrobial effect to regular waves of motility while we're fasted to sweep the contents of our small intestine ever forward and prevent the bacteria from getting too comfortable and settling in for the long haul. This is for good reason: The small intestine is where most nutrient digestion and absorption takes place. Having too much bacteria around all that yet-to-be-absorbed food means that some of the nutrients we ingest will be diverted to these hungry bacteria instead of being available entirely for our own use.

But there are a variety of reasons that the guardrails against excessive bacteria in the small intestine may fail—see Table 6-1 for some risk factors worth discussing with your doctor. When this happens, you may wind up with overgrowth of these bacteria. We call it overgrowth rather than an infection, because these bacteria are not necessarily disease-causing invaders. Rather, they are members of our own gut microbiota that don't normally cause harm when they're staying put in the mouth or the colon where they most belong. I've heard doctors compare bacterial overgrowth to weeds in the garden; which is to say, they are usually benign when interspersed in a diverse meadow and kept in check by many other plant species, but they can wreak havoc when they gain a foothold in your flower beds and start to take over. The bacteria most commonly implicated in SIBO are the weed-like species from the *E. coli* and *Klebsiella* genera (that's plural for *genus*, a categorization that groups related bacterial species), but it is not unheard of for people to overgrow bacteria from species that we typically think of as beneficial, including *Lactobacillus*.

Having excess bacteria in the small intestine can contribute to malabsorption of fat and/or bile acid diarrhea in some people. This is because large populations of bacteria that encounter the digestive fluid bile—often before it has the opportunity to do its job in aiding fat digestion—will modify it in a process called deconjugation. Breaking down the bile may prevent some fat and fat-soluble vitamins like vitamins A, D, E, and K from being absorbed. Unintended weight loss, deficiencies of any of these vitamins, and/or increased fat in the stool—which you may recognize as oily stools or stools that float—may therefore result from SIBO. And modification of these bile acids too early in the digestive process makes them unrecyclable, possibly contributing to bile acid diarrhea. (See the section above on bile acid diarrhea if you missed this explanation.) It's worth noting that diarrhea is seldom the only presenting symptom

Table 6-1: Common Reasons for Developing SIBO

Post-Infectious	Characteristic disruptions in the small intestine's bacterial ecosystem that commonly develop in the aftermath of food poisoning or bacterial gastroenteritis
Structural or Anatomical Abnormalities Affecting the Small Intestine	Intestinal surgeries where the valve separating the small intestine and colon has been removed (ileocecal valve)
	Presence of little herniations (pouches or pockets), called diverticula, in the small intestine
	Weight loss surgeries such as the Roux-en-Y gastric bypass procedure
Low Stomach Acid	Atrophic or autoimmune gastritis that reduces stomach acid secretion
	Chronic use of proton pump inhibitor (PPI) medications
	Long-standing infection with *H. pylori* bacteria (?)
Slow or Impaired Motility in the Small Intestine	Medications that slow down intestinal transit time (narcotic painkillers, anticholinergic medications for diarrhea)
	Scar tissue or adhesions around the intestine from prior abdominal surgeries
	Slow motility in the small intestine (may be primarily caused by hypothyroidism, connective tissue diseases, Sjögren's syndrome)
	Strictures (narrowing) in the small intestine due to Crohn's disease
Inflammation in the Small Intestine	Inflammation in the ileum (ileitis) from Crohn's disease or excess use of over-the-counter pain medications (NSAIDs)
	Undiagnosed or poorly managed celiac disease
Low Levels of Pancreatic Fluids	Exocrine pancreatic insufficiency (EPI)
Other	Chronic alcohol overuse
	End-stage kidney disease

of SIBO; often people will experience one or more other issues, including significant gas and bloating following certain meals, abdominal pain, acid reflux, nausea, and even brain fog. Those people who overgrow an organism called *Methanobrevibacter smithii* may actually experience constipation instead of diarrhea as their primary SIBO symptom. The constipation is directly caused by the methane gas that these organisms produce, and is sometimes called methanogenic SIBO or methane-predominant SIBO.

SIBO VERSUS METHANE OVERGROWTH

In recognition of the fact that having higher levels of methane gas in the gut can be constipating, the existence of a sister condition to SIBO called intestinal methane overgrowth (IMO) has been proposed. The difference between methane-predominant SIBO and IMO has to do with where the methane is actually being produced. IMO would refer to having high levels of methane-producing organisms in the colon, even if they are not necessarily overgrowing in the small intestine as would be the case in SIBO.

Because of the constipating effect of methane gas, it is increasingly recognized that harboring even normal amounts of methane-producing organisms in the colon might still pose a problem for some. Referring back to our gardening analogy: Just like a lawn needs to be weeded from time to time, it has been proposed that people with IMO may require periodic courses of specific antibiotics that target archaea—the methane-producing organisms—to suppress their ranks. Experimental studies of a common cholesterol-lowering drug called lovastatin lactone suggested it might be an effective way to treat constipation due to methane overgrowth for people with constipation-predominant irritable bowel syndrome (IBS-C) by inhibiting methane production, but later-phase clinical trials in 2020 failed to live up to the promising early results. It remains to be seen whether this medication will be explored as a potential adjunctive treatment for methane-predominant SIBO.

How Do Symptoms of SIBO Present?

One of the most common complaints associated with SIBO is bloating, which is both excess gas (usually farting, but sometimes burping) as well as a significantly distended belly compared with what's normal for you. Mornings are usually the best time of the day, digestively speaking, with gas and bloating building as the day progresses and you eat a variety of foods. Often, certain foods will trigger acute gas, bloating, and/or diarrhea within thirty to sixty minutes of eating them, even if these are foods you used to eat all the time without any trouble. Most commonly, foods high in families of carbohydrates called FODMAPs will trigger these symptoms (see Table 4-1 in Chapter 4 for a list), but for some people, foods high in sugar, starches/carbs, or fat will set off symptoms, too. The gas and bloating can be quite painful, and many people experience significant abdominal discomfort or pain.

Most people with SIBO also experience a change in their bathroom patterns and stool consistency, though this can take many forms. Some people experience diarrhea, more frequent bowel movements, more urgent bowel movements, and/or strangely colored or textured stools. Stool might be lighter colored than normal, oilier, stickier/harder to wipe, looser, and/or it may feel acidic on its way out. However, some people with SIBO can become suddenly quite constipated. How SIBO affects your bowel movements often correlates to the type of organisms you are overgrowing and the type of gas they produce as described in the previous section.

Other symptoms associated with SIBO include acid reflux; nausea; unexplained vitamin B_{12} deficiency; feelings of brain fog (forgetfulness, cloudy thinking); and/or weight changes.

Diagnosing SIBO

In research settings, diagnosing SIBO had once involved taking a sample of fluid from your small intestine and analyzing its bacterial load. This is an invasive process—and not necessarily without its own limitations in terms of false-positive and false-negative results. As a result, it is far more common for SIBO to be diagnosed with a less invasive test that uses breath gases as a proxy for bacterial populations in the gut rather than measuring the bacterial populations directly. **Breath testing** measures changes in your breath gases in response to consuming sugars that bacteria typically love to ferment.

The premise of breath testing goes like this: There are certain gases that only bacteria produce. So if we can measure these gases on your breath, we know that bacteria made them. Knowing what we know about how long it takes for liquids to travel from the mouth, through the stomach, into the small intestine, and finally arrive to the colon, we can approximate where in the digestive system bacterial fermentation of sugar is taking place based on how long after drinking the sugar solution the post-fermentation gases appear on your breath. (Pretty clever, right?)

The simple test involves you showing up fasted, breathing into a bag to provide a baseline measurement of the gases on your breath, drinking some sugar water, and then breathing into a bag every fifteen to twenty minutes for three hours. The technician will feed each breath sample into a special machine that measures concentration of hydrogen and methane gases. Mail-away test kits are also available to people who don't live near a gastroenterology practice that administers the test in person, though the quality of the tests and protocols used for interpretation vary widely depending by lab. Some are very reliable while others are not.

So why is this simple, noninvasive, perfectly safe test sometimes regarded with skepticism by doctors as far as its diagnostic helpfulness? Because there are a lot of factors that can affect breath test results, making them prone to both false negatives and false positives. Many of these factors are preventable with a good pretest preparation protocol—like making sure you haven't recently had a colonoscopy and/or taken antibiotics, probiotics, or medications that affect your bowel's motility. Controlling your diet the day before the test can also ensure you don't have high amounts of gas on your breath before the test even starts. But other factors that may affect the reliability of the test results aren't necessarily known in advance and therefore can't be controlled. For example, since breath testing assumes you have normal transit time of liquids throughout the digestive tract, anyone with an undiagnosed motility problem—especially slow stomach emptying or a sluggish small intestine—may be at risk of a false negative. A less common cause of false negatives relates to our lack of precise knowledge about what types of bacteria a given person might be overgrowing. In my clinical practice, we've occasionally encountered patients who tested negative for SIBO when given the usual sugar solutions—glucose or lactose—only to later learn that they were overgrowing a somewhat unusual type of bacteria that preferentially likes to ferment fructose or lactose sugar. The SIBO only showed up once we administered a fructose or lactose breath test in search of a different diagnosis of dietary fructose or lactose intolerance (see Chapter 5 for more on these conditions).

The nontrivial rates of false positives and negatives associated with breath testing have led many doctors to dismiss the test's utility entirely. I've encountered numerous patients whose doctors "don't believe in" the test, and will simply prescribe antibiotics to any patient whom they suspect *might* have SIBO. Sometimes the gamble pays off and my patients improve. Other times, a patient's symptoms do not resolve after a course of antibiotics prescribed on a hunch. This introduces a quandary: Was the lack of response a sign that the patient didn't have SIBO to begin with? Or could it mean that they did have SIBO, but the antibiotic selected simply didn't eradicate the particular critters the patient was overgrowing? The most recent data available suggest that only about 50% of confirmed SIBO cases resolve after the first course of antibiotics prescribed, so if we had data from a breath test that strongly suggested SIBO, a lack of response to the first antibiotic of choice might lead a doctor to try re-treating, possibly with a different medication. Without data from an albeit imperfect breath test to validate the diagnostic hunch, it's common for doctors to assume that the problem must not have been SIBO and land on a diagnosis of irritable bowel syndrome (IBS) (see Chapters 4, 10).

While we recognize the possibility of false positives or negatives inherent to breath testing in our clinical practice, we nonetheless believe strongly in the utility of testing as providing an additional data point for consideration in the diagnostic journey. As the saying goes, "Don't make perfect the enemy of good." Just because a test doesn't deliver 100% perfect results 100% of the time, that doesn't mean it has no place in clinical practice. Even breath test data that are somewhat equivocal—not a clear-cut negative or positive—can be considered alongside other important clues to help sway the gastroenterologist's clinical judgment in favor of or against a diagnosis of SIBO. And we take good care to prep our breath test patients well and administer a test that meets the most recent consensus-based protocols for the test itself and the interpretation of results, which increases the likelihood of deriving meaningful data from it. More data are better than fewer, and so our practice's philosophy is quite in favor of breath testing—at least for now. In our gastroenterology practice, we are looking forward to the commercialization of a swallowable diagnostic capsule currently under development that may be able to provide much more accurate counts of intestinal bacterial loads for more precise SIBO diagnoses.

Stool tests, including stool microbiome analyses, are *absolutely not* a scientifically validated way to diagnose SIBO. The fecal microbiota—or the community of microorganisms present in your stool—is vastly different from the small intestinal microbiota. You cannot draw any conclusions whatsoever about which organisms are living in your small intestine and at what levels based on an analysis of your stool. Nor can you draw conclusions about small intestinal bacterial loads by examining other features of the stool, including the stool's pH or presence of other organic compounds. Anyone who claims they can diagnose SIBO based on a stool analysis is not practicing evidence-based medicine, and, in my experience, is likely trying to sell you supplements.

Treating SIBO

As of the time of this writing, broad-spectrum, prescription antibiotics are the only evidence-based treatment for eradicating SIBO. Broad-spectrum antibiotics are those that can kill members of the two main classifications of bacteria—gram-positive bacteria and gram-negative bacteria. This is important because currently available breath tests can't actually tell us what specific species or strains of bacteria you are overgrowing in the small bowel so as to inform a very tailored choice of medication. It is common for a medication called rifaximin (Xifaxan) to be prescribed as a first-line treatment, since it's not absorbed into the body from the gut, though its success rate is not necessarily superior to the many other broad-spectrum antibiotic choices available to your doctor. As mentioned earlier, the success rate of treatment with a single course of antibiotics is about 50%, so it's pretty common for people to require a second course of this drug or a different medication if their symptoms do not resolve the first time around.

Patients who are found to have both hydrogen and methane gas on their breath test may be prescribed rifaximin (or a different broad-spectrum antibiotic) plus a second antibiotic like neomycin or metronidazole (Flagyl) since the type of organisms that produce methane gas aren't typically affected by rifaximin alone. These medications are most effective when taken at the same time rather than sequentially. If your symptoms do not respond to the first choice of an antibiotic, it is common for doctors to prescribe a different medication, and the drug decision may be based on factors such as cost, allergies you may have to certain antibiotics, and/or past experience with side effects from specific medications.

While many other SIBO protocols involving some combination of elimination diets, probiotics, herbal essential oil extracts, and other purported "herbal antimicrobials" abound, none of these have been appropriately tested and validated as effective treatments for SIBO. People who are steeped in the world of SIBO or who practice functional/integrative medicine often refer to a 2014 study that claimed equivalence of herbal remedies to the prescription antibiotic rifaximin to justify the use of such alternative medicine regimens. A closer reading of this often-cited study, however, reveals that the authors used nonstandard, laxer criteria for diagnosing SIBO, raising the question as to how many of the study's participants even had SIBO to begin with. The dose of rifaximin used in the study was lower than the standard dose used to treat SIBO in the real world, meaning that patients were undermedicated with antibiotics. Furthermore, results of the analysis on which basis the authors claimed that herbals were as effective as a prescription antibiotic were not statistically significant, since there were only seventeen patients who seemed to improve on herbal regimens. This essentially means that there is a very low chance that the results of this study would be replicated in a larger population of people with SIBO if this study were to be repeated (and, I suppose, if the participants even actually had SIBO to begin with). Long story short: The only evidence we have in support of the efficacy of herbal remedies to treat SIBO isn't actually very good evidence that herbals treat SIBO at all, and certainly not as well as a standard dose of an antibiotic tailored to the type of SIBO a person has. It's important to read past headlines and into the fine print, especially since these herbal regimens typically cost hundreds of dollars, are not covered by insurance, and when they don't work, can wind up delaying effective treatment for many months.

With regard to the question of probiotics and SIBO, most anything you read about whether they're helpful or harmful is based on opinion, not evidence. There are scant actual scientific data that even investigates the role of probiotic supplements and SIBO: Can they help treat it or prevent it? Might they actually cause it or make it worse? I've seen one or two tiny studies that suggest the former, and an equal number that suggest the latter. The bottom line is that the question hasn't been investigated thoroughly enough to say for sure.

In my clinical practice, I advise my patients with SIBO to avoid taking any bacterial probiotics either during or after their treatment. Since SIBO can sometimes actually involve the over-growth of benign—or even beneficial—species/strains of bacteria in a region of the digestive tract whose fail-safes to prevent this occurrence have, well, failed . . . it concerns me to have my patients introducing concentrated pills full of more bacteria into that environment. Part of me wonders (worries?) whether people who continue to experience recurrences of SIBO one after another might be unwittingly repopulating their own susceptible small intestine with probiotic supplements that deliver their contents too early in the digestive journey. If stronger evidence emerges to support the use of specific probiotics in the treatment or prevention of SIBO, I will happily change my tune. Until that time, I do not object to my patients taking yeast-based probiotics, such as various *Saccharomyces boulardii* strains, if they are so inclined to try a probiotic.

Dietary Management of SIBO

Diet can play a helpful role in managing the severity of symptoms when you have SIBO. Avoiding certain foods has not been shown to cure SIBO, nor has consuming certain foods been shown to cause SIBO, with the notable exception of excess alcohol consumption. As such, in my clinical opinion, whether you change your diet or not when SIBO is suspected or diagnosed is a decision that should be based entirely on quality-of-life issues. If the inconvenience of restricting your diet is outweighed by the symptom relief it brings you, then it may be worth it. Most of my patients do choose to avoid certain foods when they have untreated SIBO. But ideally, I try to have them restrict their diets for the minimum time required between suspicion for, diagnosis of, and treatment of their SIBO—for a matter of weeks, not months, and especially not years.

There is almost no research to support which diet(s) are best for managing symptoms of SIBO, though the most common and least restrictive approach by far is the **low-FODMAP diet**. FODMAP is an acronym for

Fermentable *(a scientific way of saying that bacteria can break it down and make gas)*

Oligosaccharides *(refers to a variety of poorly digested carbohydrates found in certain grains, beans, and veggies)*

Disaccharides *(in this case, it refers to a sugar called lactose)*

Monosaccharides *(in this case, it refers to a sugar called fructose)*

And

Polyols *(also known as "sugar alcohols," any sugar whose name ends with the suffix -ol)*

See Chapter 4, pages 55–62, for a more detailed description of the low-FODMAP diet and food lists.

Consuming only foods that do not contain any of these fermentable carbohydrates or sugars can help manage symptoms of SIBO until it's been successfully eradicated. I often encounter patients whose doctors advise them to start a low-FODMAP diet *after* completing treatment for SIBO, and this recommendation has never made much sense to me. If ever there was going to be a time that a person who's been suffering the effects of SIBO could safely and comfortably enjoy high-FODMAP foods like beans, cauliflower, or watermelon ... wouldn't it be immediately after the gas-producing members of the gut microbiome have had their ranks suppressed by a course of antibiotics? Since there is no evidence to support the notion that consuming a FODMAP-containing diet causes SIBO, I fail to see the case for ongoing diet restriction after treatment has been completed—especially if your symptoms suggest that treatment has been successful. Furthermore, we know that diverse, high-fiber diets support abundant, healthy, diverse, and resilient gut microbiomes, suggesting that prolonged adherence to symptom-managing but microbiota-starving low-FODMAP diets may not be in the best interest of long-term gut health. For these reasons, I encourage my patients to focus their energy on working with their doctor to help isolate the reason they developed SIBO to begin with so as to reduce the risk of a recurrence if possible rather than remain on restricted diets indefinitely.

There are other diets you may encounter online that are sometimes used in combination with or instead of the low-FODMAP diet. These include the specific carbohydrate diet, or SCD, which essentially eliminates all sugars, grains, and starchy/root vegetables—even those that are low-FODMAP—in addition to most beans/legumes that are already prohibited on the low-FODMAP diet. The SCD does allow many high-FODMAP vegetables and fruits, however, which aren't necessarily going to be well tolerated in people with SIBO. There are therefore hybrid versions of the low-FODMAP diet and SCD circulating online—often referred to as SIBO diets or the biphasic diet—that restrict all grains, starches, and sugars plus high-FODMAP fruits, veggies, and nuts. These should almost certainly help with symptom control among people with SIBO but may be far more restrictive than necessary. Many people find that avoiding high-FODMAP foods alone is plenty effective to manage their diarrhea and other symptoms without having to also avoid foods like rice, potatoes, a little bit of sugar, or lactose-free milk.

Celiac Disease

Celiac disease is an autoimmune disease in which the body's immune cells launch a self-directed attack against the lining of the small intestine in response to ingestion of a **protein** called **gluten**, found in wheat, barley, rye, and other foods that may have come into cross contact with them. It is a hereditary disease, which means that with very few exceptions, people must carry at least one of the two genes that predispose to celiac disease in order to develop the condition. But having the celiac gene(s) does not guarantee you will eventually develop the condition; in fact, while an estimated 40% of Caucasians carry at least one of the genes associated with celiac disease, only about 1% of Americans actually have celiac disease. White Americans and people with Punjabi ancestry are more likely to develop celiac disease than people with Hispanic, non-Hispanic, Black, and East Asian heritage, though there is some question about whether disparities in healthcare across races may result in underdiagnosis of celiac disease in nonwhite people. Whites with Irish or Scandinavian ancestry may be at even higher risk. However, humans are beautifully complex and there are often unknown relationships in our family trees that contribute to our genetic makeup, so you can't say for sure that you couldn't have celiac disease based solely on your identification with a lower-risk group.

Researchers have been making progress about determining what sets off celiac disease in someone who is genetically at risk for it. Our current understanding suggests that disease onset probably involves a perfect storm of biological and environmental factors happening all at once. Specifically, developing celiac disease may involve having impaired barrier function of the mucous lining of the gut that allows fragments of gluten protein to slip into the deeper layers of the gut wall and interact with immune cells. This impaired barrier function—often referred to as intestinal permeability or gut leakiness—can occur in the aftermath of a viral infection or under other circumstances, and may be worsened by having low vitamin D levels. More research is needed to refine the details of this hypothesis.

When someone with celiac disease ingests even the most minute amount of gluten, it activates immune cells embedded in the gut tissue. These immune cells quickly mobilize an inflammatory response that winds up damaging the intestines. The inflammatory response doesn't necessarily turn off when, say, the offending mouthful of gluten-containing food has exited the small intestine and its residue pooped out. Rather, it can linger on for some time, causing more damage to the gut's absorptive lining than would be expected from such a tiny bit of gluten exposure. And when gluten consumption occurs consistently in someone with celiac disease— whether by accident or due to semi-regular intentional cheats on the gluten-free diet—it can result in significant-enough damage to the small intestine's lining as to affect nutrient absorption. In fact, some of the more common signs of undiagnosed celiac disease are iron deficiency anemia and early-onset osteoporosis, due to chronic iron and calcium malabsorption, respectively. Other nutritional deficiencies, unintended weight loss, and infertility and miscarriages in women are other potential outcomes from undiagnosed or poorly managed celiac disease.

Celiac disease is not considered a gluten allergy, simply because the body's response to gluten is not mediated by the same type of immune cells as a typical food allergy is.

How Do Symptoms of Celiac Disease Present?

Diarrhea is the most common presenting symptom of celiac disease in adults, whereas abdominal pain is actually more common among children. But not everyone with celiac disease experiences diarrhea. Some may actually experience constipation, and others may have no change at all in their bowel movements. Bloating, gas, and abdominal pain are other common gastrointestinal complaints associated with celiac disease, though it's also possible to have no digestive symptoms at all. I often hear that the type of belly distension produced when someone with celiac disease consumes wheat or gluten-containing foods can resemble an inflated balloon and last for several days. It can often be quite painful and even debilitating.

Some people experience joint pain or aches, headaches, fatigue, or skin rashes. Conversely, some people with silent celiac disease may have no symptoms whatsoever. The disease is only found when doctors start investigating the possible reason behind other ailments, such as iron deficiency anemia, osteoporosis, SIBO, or unintended weight loss. Such nutritional deficiencies are a common feature of celiac disease.

For most people who have diarrhea as a presenting symptom of celiac disease, the diarrhea should begin to subside within several weeks on a gluten-free diet. If it persists, the first step is to have a qualified registered dietitian take a look at your diet to ensure it is as strictly gluten-free as you think it is. If there is truly no cause to think you're having ongoing gluten exposure, it may be prudent to consider the possibility of other concurrent conditions. People with as-yet-undiagnosed celiac disease are at elevated risk for developing

SIBO (see previous section of this chapter), and even when you go gluten-free to address the celiac disease–related inflammation, the overgrowing bacteria aren't budging. Another possibility is that you have concurrently developed irritable bowel syndrome (Chapter 4); one study of 1,000 people with well-controlled celiac disease found that 23% of them met the criteria for also having IBS! In the early stages post-diagnosis, you may also experience gas and diarrhea from a temporary form of lactose intolerance (Chapter 5) caused by damage to the lactase-enzyme-producing tips of your intestinal cells. This should resolve with time as the celiac-related inflammation recedes and the gut has time to repair itself.

Diagnosing Celiac Disease

In order to obtain an accurate diagnosis of celiac disease, you'll need to have been eating foods that contain gluten regularly for several weeks prior to testing—ideally six. There is little point in being tested for celiac disease if you've been following a gluten-free diet for any extended period of time, as the risk of false-negative results is high.

Diagnosis is typically a two-step process. Blood work is the first step, and your doctor will likely order a celiac panel, which includes measurements of several antibodies. Specifically, a celiac panel involves checking anti-transglutaminase (or anti-tTg) antibodies. It also checks total levels of IgA antibodies to ensure your immune system functions properly enough to actually mount an antibody response if you did have celiac disease and prevent the possibility of a false-negative result. People who are deficient in IgA antibodies should be given additional blood tests to measure deamidated gliadin peptide (DGP) antibodies and/or a different type of anti-tTg antibodies from the IgG antibody class.

If there are elevated blood markers suggesting that celiac disease is a possibility, a gastroenterologist will need to perform an upper endoscopy in order to take biopsies (tissue samples) of the first segment of your small intestine (duodenum) to look for tell-tale signs of the inflammation and damage caused by celiac disease. Because celiac disease activity can be patchy, it is a best practice for doctors to take multiple biopsies from different places so as to reduce the risk of false-negative results; six or more are commonly taken in our practice. I can recall a patient I once saw with a genetic risk factor (Irish heritage) and all the telltale signs of celiac disease—diarrhea, weight loss, iron deficiency, and a new-onset lactose intolerance. He was told that he didn't have celiac disease based on an endoscopy where only a single biopsy was taken. Skeptical, I recommended the gluten-free diet anyway, and the symptoms resolved, suggesting strongly that he had received a false-negative result.

Treating Celiac Disease

A strict gluten-free diet for life is the only known treatment for celiac disease that we have at present. How strict is strict enough? The best data we have available suggests that anything over 10 mg of gluten could provoke an immune response in most people with celiac disease, though even lower levels can be problematic for extremely sensitive individuals. As a visual, 10 mg of gluten would roughly resemble the crumbs left on a plate after finishing a piece of toast. This means that people with celiac disease have to avoid foods that overtly contain gluten from wheat, barley, or rye-derived ingredients, and they also must take great care to ensure their gluten-free food has not had cross contact with gluten-containing foods such that crumbs or flour could accidentally make it into their meal—and mouths. In a home where some household members consume gluten and others have celiac disease, shared sticks of butter or peanut butter jars where double-dipping takes place, shared pop-up toasters, and porous wooden cutting boards used for bread slicing or flouring are all potential areas in which cross contamination can occur.

Someone with celiac disease who follows a strict gluten-free diet can expect to experience complete healing of their damaged intestines over several months to a year following adoption of the diet. In other words, a doctor performing endoscopy to examine your intestinal lining would not be able to tell the difference between the tissue of someone with well-controlled celiac disease (or quiescent celiac disease) compared with that of a healthy control. I mention this because many of my patients with even quiescent celiac disease seem to be under the impression that they have lots of chronic inflammation just by virtue of having this diagnosis, or that they need to adopt various supplement or dietary regimens to "heal their gut." Just to be clear: maintaining a strict gluten-free diet should quash all celiac-associated inflammation and heal the gut entirely without the need to drink bone broth, take probiotics, or spend money on any of the faddish gut-directed therapies conjured up by opportunistic marketers online.

Speaking of opportunistic marketers, there are many out there who make claims about gluten content of products or gluten digestion that are dangerous for people with celiac disease. No enzyme supplements or medications can make gluten consumption safe for people with celiac disease, period. I'm thinking specifically about DPP-IV—dipeptidyl peptidase IV—or what some marketers have dubbed glutenase, which is a supplement marketed as aiding in gluten digestion. It does NOT make gluten consumption safe for people with celiac disease, so don't believe the hype. And for the record: there is no such human digestive enzyme as glutenase.

There is also a myth that sourdough fermentation of dough removes the gluten and makes it safe for people with celiac disease. It doesn't. Neither, for that matter, does sprouting gluten-containing grains before baking them into bread. Similarly, I've seen wheat-based breads marketed as having "reduced gluten," and wheat flour–based banana breads marketed as "gluten-neutralized," whatever on God's good earth that's supposed to mean. I'm not exactly sure who the target customers for these products are, but if you have celiac disease, they're certainly NOT for you.

Dietary Management of Celiac Disease

The popularity of gluten-free diets among far more Americans than those with celiac disease is a mixed blessing for people who actually do have celiac disease. On one hand, it has pushed food manufacturers and restaurants to develop a wider variety of gluten-free foods that people with celiac disease can safely enjoy. Dedicated gluten-free bakeries have sprung up all over the place so that people with celiac disease no longer need to be deprived of bagels, birthday cakes, and other special treats, and large supermarket chains carry a variety of convenience products so that people with celiac disease can "bread" their chicken cutlets, pop a frozen dinner in the microwave, or find a suitably crunchy salty snack to munch on while bingeing Netflix shows. Ask any older person with celiac disease whether they preferred their food options twenty years ago (when no one had even heard of gluten) or now, and my guess is that they'd say living with celiac disease has never been easier than it is today.

But as more and more food manufacturers, cafés, and restaurants hop on the trendy gluten-free bandwagon to suit the preferences of wellness-oriented consumers more than the actual medical needs of the celiac community, quality control has become a huge and menacing issue. A popular bakery-café chain offers an amazing-looking, wholesome gluten-free bread that is baked in the same flour-strewn kitchen as all its other artisan breads, and sliced on the same bread-crumb-strewn counter as they are, too. Local coffee shops offer gluten-free muffins and cookies cuddled up on the same trays and nestled under the same cloches as the standard flour-based options. Many Italian restaurants now offer gluten-free pastas—but how many of them are cooking those pastas in the same pot of boiling water as the conventional wheat-based pasta? And how many gluten-free pizzas are being prepared on the same flour-strewn counters, sharing the same oven with regular pizzas without a layer of foil underneath, or cut with the same pizza slicers that were just dragged through a regular pizza five minutes prior? It can be so tempting for someone with celiac disease to partake in all these yummy-looking gluten-free options increasingly available in the world, but avoiding cross contamination can be especially tricky as these options abound.

I don't mean to give the impression that people with celiac disease should be so paranoid about gluten exposure that it would be best to cook all your own food from scratch, never eat out, or avoid travel. Virtually all my patients with celiac disease rely on packaged convenience foods, have learned how to dine out safely, and, with enough advance research and preparation, are able to partake of delicious and safe foods when they travel, too. But the key is maintaining a high degree of vigilance, asking a lot of questions, researching in advance whenever possible, and having backup plans (read: snacks on your person) in case you find yourself in a situation where gluten-free food is not available. Traveling to major cities in countries in which prevalence of celiac disease is high and waitstaff speak English—like Ireland and Sweden—is a wonderful way to get your travel feet wet as someone with celiac disease who hasn't yet taken their gluten-free diet on the road. I still dream about all the delicious gluten-free foods I ate on a trip to Stockholm—including reindeer meatballs! Mexico and Central America are also extremely easy places for people with celiac disease to travel, as naturally gluten-free staples like corn, beans, and rice form the basis of the local cuisines, and flour/wheat are not typically used in sauces.

And then there's the issue with misleading ingredient labels on packaged food. Rule No. 1 for following a gluten-free diet is never relying solely on gluten-free label callouts on packaged foods as a green light without actually reading ingredient lists. This is for a few reasons. For starters, US law does not require product manufacturers to test their products and verify they are gluten-free before using a "gluten-free" label claim. Rather, regulations allow use of the claim for any food product that is not manufactured with wheat, barley, rye, or ingredients derived from them. Seems reasonable enough, right? The problem is that this regulation allows for a huge loophole: It allows products using any old kind of oats to legally make a "gluten-free" claim despite the well-known high risk of gluten contamination of conventionally processed oats. Between growing, sorting, and processing, oats are rather likely to come into contact with stray grains of wheat and barley that went through the same storage containers or machinery, and errant gluten-containing grains can find their way into batches of oats that are grown, harvested, transported, sorted, milled, and/or packaged in shared spaces. Therefore, products that contain conventionally processed oats do have the potential to be cross-contaminated with gluten—and testing from the Gluten Free Watchdog, an independent, subscription-based, product-testing service run by registered dietitian Tricia Thompson, confirms that they commonly are. Thompson recommends choosing only oat products that have come to market via a "purity protocol" that takes extra precautions to keep oats away from gluten-containing grains throughout all steps of the process, as well as those gluten-free oats sorted via the technique employed by Quaker Oats. You can view a list of products that contain purity protocol oats that meet Thompson's stringent standards by visiting her website at www.glutenfreewatchdog.org/.

Another issue with relying solely on gluten-free label claims pertains to mislabeling of gluten-free products, which is rampant among packaged foods. You'd be shocked to learn how many products on supermarket shelves carry a "gluten-free" shout-out on the front of the package while listing gluten-containing ingredients like wheat-based soy sauce, malt flavoring, or even wheat flour on the back of the package. People with celiac disease must therefore get into the habit of ignoring label claims and reading the entire list of ingredients to ensure a product's suitability, and to do so each time they purchase a different product even from brands they have come to know and trust.

If you have celiac disease and this seems daunting to you, I'd suggest acquainting yourself further with the writing and advocacy of Tricia Thompson, MS, RD, who I introduced a few paragraphs ago. She's been involved in the tireless and often thankless work of spotting misbranded, mislabeled products and bringing them to the attention of manufacturers, the FDA, and the public; auditing random "gluten-free" labeled products by having their gluten content verified by independent lab testing; and stress-testing the reliability of oat-based products that claim to be gluten-free based on newer grain-sorting methods rather than the more established purity protocols. Tricia's sleuthing has brought to light gluten-free labeling errors among large potato chip brands that contain malt flavoring (derived from barley); gluten-free baking mixes that list wheat flour in their ingredients; and a variety of Asian condiments and packaged meals labeled "gluten-free" that contain soy sauce that's derived from wheat.

WORDS ON A NUTRITION LABEL
THAT IMPLY GLUTEN

Barley	Oats*
Bread crumbs	Orzo
Bulgur	Pastry flour
Couscous	Pumpernickel
Durum wheat	Rye
Einkorn	Semolina
Enriched flour	Soy sauce (tamari is OK)
Flour	Spelt
Kamut	Texturized vegetable
Macaroni	protein (TVP)
Malt flavoring, barley malt	Triticale
Matzah or matzo meal	Wheat
Miso (often barley based)	

* Look for "gluten-free oats" to ensure safety from cross contamination

Learning how to scrutinize ingredient labels is an important skill to learn as a person with celiac disease, and ideally you should try to find a local registered dietitian who has ample experience with celiac disease to teach you the tricks of the trade. If you don't have access to someone with the right credentials and expertise, the next best thing would be to invest in Shelley Case's authoritative book, *Gluten Free: The Definitive Resource Guide*. Case is a Canadian registered dietitian who has encyclopedic knowledge of the gluten-free diet. Her book is an exhaustive reference on eating, grocery shopping, dining out, traveling, and drinking alcohol safely when you have celiac disease. It's really a must-have for anyone with, celiac disease—or anyone who lives with, cooks for, travels with, or simply just loves someone with celiac disease.

Another important aspect of your diet to vet for gluten content is your medication and dietary supplement regimen. It is exceedingly common for dietary supplements to contain wheat-derived fillers or coatings, and disturbingly common for these ingredients to be undeclared or unlabeled. In the United States, dietary supplements are so laxly regulated that product marketers don't have to prove that their supplements actually contain what they say they do (or don't contain what they say they don't) before placing said products on store shelves. Audits of randomly selected products conducted by various parties—from state attorneys general to subscription-based supplement review services—routinely uncover evidence of products that contain undeclared ingredients, and among them wheat is a more common one. I can't tell you how many patients with celiac disease I've counseled who presented to me with worsening digestive symptoms despite extreme vigilance with their gluten-free diet. A blood test verified that their celiac disease was active again. But where was the gluten exposure coming from? In all these cases, the symptoms began a few months after consulting functional/integrative medicine practitioners who put them on extensive dietary supplement regimens. Even though each and every one of the more than a dozen supplements was labeled "gluten-free," clearly at least one of them was carrying some unde-clared wheat ingredients. When the supplementation stops, the symptoms improve soon after, and within a few months, the celiac antibody markers return to normal.

My takeaway? When you have celiac disease, the fewer dietary supplements you take, the better. When there is a need for a sup-plement, choose large, US-based brands that are likely to own their own manufacturing facilities and can afford internal quality con-trol departments. Smaller, boutique supplement brands are far more likely to outsource their supplement production to third-party man-ufacturers in China, where quality control standards are known to be lax. I also recommend seeking out supplement products that bear the "USP Verified" logo. The United States Pharmacopeia (USP) is a nonprofit group that offers third-party verification of the qual-ity of dietary supplements, testing that (1) products contain what they say they do; (2) products aren't contaminated with harmful ingredients, like heavy metals or undeclared drugs; and (3) prod-ucts are manufactured according to good manufacturing practices. While there are no complete guarantees, a product that has passed USP verification is probably less likely to harbor undeclared glu-ten from messy manufacturing cross contact or as a filler to replace more expensive active ingredients.

Undeclared gluten should be less of a problem with both pre-scription and over-the-counter medications, as these categories of products are subject to more regulatory scrutiny from are dietary supplements. Still, anytime you are prescribed a new medication or your pharmacist replaces your usual medication with a generic alternative manufactured somewhere different from your usual, you should ask the pharmacist to check the product's inactive ingredi-ents to ensure they are all gluten-free.

Finally, even as you adapt to your gluten-free diet and feel as though you have everything under control, it's important to follow up annually with your primary care doctor or gastroenterologist for surveillance. Having your celiac antibody levels checked annually—along with iron levels and other basic nutrition labs—is a good habit to get into to verify that your diet is as gluten-free as you thought it was and is keeping the inflammation at bay. Talk to your doctor about other onetime or routine healthcare maintenance that may be required on the basis of your new celiac disease diagnosis. Some patients are advised to have a baseline bone density scan (DEXA scan) taken to evaluate whether there have been bone density losses as the result of prior calcium malabsorption from the celiac disease pre-diagnosis. Patients with celiac disease are also advised to get pneumonia vaccinations every five years, even if they are under age sixty-five.

Some people with celiac disease may experience ongoing digestive symptoms—including persistent diarrhea, gas, and bloating—even after adopting a gluten-free diet in response to their celiac disease diagnosis. In these cases, we first look at your diet to ensure it is indeed as gluten-free as you believe it to be; ongoing intake due to hidden gluten in beverages, supplements or confections is not uncommon. However, when your diet is truly, strictly, and completely gluten-free, then we need to consider other possibilities.

In my practice, there's a high index of suspicion for SIBO (see previous section) in our patients with newly diagnosed celiac disease whose symptoms are not adequately improving on a gluten-free diet. This is because uncontrolled celiac disease is associated with increased risk of developing SIBO. If you developed SIBO before your celiac disease was diagnosed, you will still have that SIBO even as you treat the celiac disease with a gluten-free diet. Fortunately, if this is the case, once you eradicate the SIBO with antibiotics, it's likely that the condition won't recur so long as you keep your celiac disease quiet with consistent adherence to your gluten-free diet.

Exocrine Pancreatic Insufficiency (EPI)

The pancreas is an accessory organ to the digestive system. One of its essential jobs is to produce key enzymes required to break down carbohydrates (amylase), proteins (protease), and fats (lipase);

it also delivers a substance called pancreatic bicarbonate that neutralizes the acidic contents arriving from the stomach. Collectively, these fluids are delivered directly into the early part of the small intestine through a dedicated duct called the pancreatic duct. Pancreatic bicarbonate has an antimicrobial effect, and therefore helps play a role in keeping the small intestine clear of excess bacteria. For this reason, a deficiency in pancreatic secretions—which is called **exocrine pancreatic insufficiency (EPI)**—is a risk factor for developing SIBO (see pages 103–115).

The lack of adequate levels of pancreatic enzymes that accompanies EPI results in malabsorption of some calorie-containing nutrients—whether carbohydrates, proteins, or fats—and this, in turn, often results in unintentional weight loss. Because our body has some backup ways to absorb carbohydrates—including sugar and starch-digesting enzymes manufactured by cells lining the small intestine—many people with pancreatic insufficiency can still do a reasonable job absorbing fat-free starchy and sweet foods like rice, bread, pasta, cereal, crackers, potatoes, fruit, and sugary things like jams, juices, or candy. Fat malabsorption is the greatest issue for people with EPI, and it is also most responsible for the signature type of diarrhea often associated with EPI.

How Do Symptoms of Exocrine Pancreatic Insufficiency Present?

Symptoms associated with EPI include substantial amounts of looser stools, which are worse following higher-fat meals. Unintentional weight loss or difficulty maintaining your weight due to incomplete calorie absorption is also a common feature, as is producing a significant amount of (often foul-smelling) gas. The diarrhea itself will often carry signs of fat malabsorption; stools may float or appear greasy and/or you may even observe oil droplets in the toilet water. Often, the color of your stool will be lighter than normal— even orangey. The type of diarrhea associated with fat malabsorption from pancreatic insufficiency has its own name: **steatorrhea**.

People with EPI may also develop deficiencies in certain vitamins that require fat to be absorbed well; these include vitamin A, vitamin E, vitamin K, and vitamin D, though since most vitamin D comes from the sun rather than from our food to begin with, a vitamin D deficiency is far more likely to represent a sunshine deficiency than a pancreatic enzyme deficiency.

Exocrine pancreatic insufficiency is often caused by chronic inflammation of the pancreas—called chronic pancreatitis. People who consume alcohol frequently and/or in larger amounts are more prone to chronic pancreatitis, though certainly alcohol overuse is not the only cause. Other conditions that can result in pancreatic insufficiency include cystic fibrosis, severe or recurrent gallstone pancreatitis, and autoimmune pancreatitis, though some otherwise healthy people simply develop it as they age. Pancreatic insufficiency can also be one of the first signs of pancreatic cancer, so it would be prudent to be screened for this if there are no other identifiable risk factors to explain your diagnosis of EPI.

Diagnosing Exocrine Pancreatic Insufficiency

Exocrine pancreatic insufficiency can be diagnosed by a simple stool test that measures levels of a marker called **elastase** in a sample of stool you send to a lab. If your stool contains less than 200 micrograms (µg) of elastase per gram of stool, you will be diagnosed with EPI, though some doctors will combine this stool test with imaging to ensure the diagnosis is reliable.

In some cases, doctors who suspect fat malabsorption as a cause for diarrhea may order a different type of stool test called a 72-hour fecal fat test, and it is as unpleasant as the name implies. You will be required to follow an extremely high-fat diet (usually 100 g per day or more, which I suppose may not bother a seasoned keto dieter), and then collect all your stool for three full days. The 72-hour collection is then submitted to a lab for analysis to measure how much of that fat ended up in your stool. A higher amount than normal would suggest fat malabsorption, though it alone is not diagnostic for EPI. A positive fecal fat test may tell us that you're malabsorbing fat, but it doesn't tell us why.

Treating Exocrine Pancreatic Insufficiency

Exocrine pancreatic insufficiency is treated with prescription enzyme supplements called pancreatic enzyme replacement therapy (PERT). These capsules often have a durable coating designed to protect the enzymes from the acid bath of the stomach and resist breaking down until arrival in the small intestine. (One brand called Viokase is uncoated and must be taken with an acid-reducing medication.) The capsules are taken along with food right at the beginning of a meal or snack so that when the capsule breaks down in the small intestine, the enzymes contained within are comingling with the food that needs to be digested and can work their biochemical magic. For longer, multicourse meals, you may even need to use some enzymes at the outset of the meal and some more partway through the meal to ensure adequate coverage. Stomach acid inactivates pancreatic enzymes, so the properly designed protective capsule is essential for them to work as intended.

Typically, you would dose your pancreatic enzymes with consideration to the amount of fat in the meal or snack. Higher-fat meals or snacks would require larger doses of pancreatic enzymes. The enzyme pills themselves are marketed at different dosage strengths, which refer to the amount of fat-digesting enzymes (lipase) they contain. People on higher-fat diets may do better with more concentrated doses of lipase so they don't need to take as many pills to adequately cover digestive needs, but dosing of enzymes is often a bit of trial and error until you land on the right number of pills for your various types of meals.

In the United States, many over-the-counter dietary supplements marketed as digestive enzyme cocktails will contain lipase as well. The doses of enzymes they list are much lower than prescription options. Because dietary supplements are minimally regulated in the United States, it's also not clear whether these products are formulated with an adequate protective coating to ensure their efficacy, or even if they actually contain the advertised dose of enzymes. In other words, if you actually have EPI, over-the-counter dietary supplement versions of digestive enzymes are a very poor substitute for prescription PERT and are not recommended.

Dietary Management of Exocrine Pancreatic Insufficiency

The main focus of dietary therapy for EPI is to consistently take your supplemental enzymes with all meals and snacks, although you do not need to use them with candy or drinks whose calories come purely from sugar, like lollipops, juice or soda. There is no need to restrict your intake of dietary fat so long as you are covering your intake adequately with enzymes; higher-fat meals or snacks will require a higher dose of enzymes than lower-fat meals, and you may need to experiment with your enzymes to get the dosing right.

Stop Drinking Alcohol

If your pancreas is already not functioning well, it is prudent to stop drinking alcohol. This is true even if your pancreatic insufficiency was not caused by alcohol use. Specialized cells in the pancreas play a role in metabolizing alcohol, and their doing so produces toxic substances and scarring as by-products. These substances can further damage the pancreas and the ducts that connect it to the digestive system to deliver enzymes. These enzymes can then build up in the pancreas and actually start digesting it, causing damage in the process and worsening its residual function.

Consider Supplementing Water-Soluble Versions of Key Vitamins

Certain dietary vitamins require fat in order to be absorbed, so if you are prone to malabsorbing fat, you are also at risk for malabsorbing these fat-soluble vitamins as well. The fat-soluble vitamins are A, D, E, and K. Pharmaceutical companies have developed modified versions of these vitamins that are water soluble and do not require fat for absorption. In the United States, you can find such a product marketed under the brand name DEKAs (Callion Pharma).

Attack of the Angry Intestines

Inflammatory Bowel Disease
(Crohn's Disease and Ulcerative Colitis)

INFLAMMATORY BOWEL DISEASE (IBD) IS a term that refers to several autoinflammatory conditions in which various segments of the gastrointestinal tract become inflamed, and often damaged, in ways that can affect nutrient absorption or the passage (motility) of food or waste. The main forms of IBD include **Crohn's disease**, which can affect any segment of the digestive tract, from mouth to anus, and **ulcerative colitis**, whose damage is limited to the colon, also known as the large intestine, and the tail end portion of the GI tract, including the rectum and anus. Both conditions can be accompanied by changes in bowel patterns—often diarrhea, but constipation is also possible; abdominal pain; blood in the stool; vitamin or mineral malabsorption and resulting deficiencies. People with IBD can also experience symptoms beyond the intestines, including mouth ulcers, fatigue, sleep disturbances, eye inflammation, skin rashes, and most commonly, joint aches and/or swelling.

To complicate matters, some of the treatments for IBD can also result in their own set of GI symptoms, even when inflammation from IBD is well controlled and is considered to be in remission. For example, when IBD cannot be adequately controlled with medications, some people require surgery to remove part or all of the affected portion of bowel. These surgeries can result in more rapid transit of food or waste through the GI tract or less intestine to do the work of digesting and absorbing, creating looser, more urgent, and more frequent stools. In other cases, such surgeries can result in internal scar tissue that adheres to the intestines, causing intestinal blockages or **obstructions** even years later. **Strictures** (narrowing of the tubular intestinal tract) may also occur as a direct result of inflammation, and these strictures can cause blockages when certain textures of fiber are consumed, especially in large quantities. When surgeries for Crohn's disease result in a removal of a segment of bowel where the small intestine and colon intersect—the ileocecal valve—it can lead to developing **small intestinal bacterial overgrowth** (SIBO; see Chapter 6), which itself may cause diarrhea, constipation, bloating, and/or food intolerances even when the IBD is in remission. Similarly, if inflammation or surgery affects the very end portion of the small intestine—called the terminal ileum—it can result in a malabsorptive type of diarrhea called **bile acid diarrhea** (see Chapter 6), which has its own set of treatments.

All of this is to say that IBD is complicated, and managing IBD symptoms can require a flexible and individualized approach, both medically and nutritionally. There is no single, standard treatment for people with IBD, nor is there a single diet for all people with IBD.

Inflammatory Bowel Disease (IBD)

Inflammatory bowel diseases like Crohn's disease and ulcerative colitis are diseases driven by one's own immune system, in which immune cells inappropriately attack healthy tissue within the digestive tract, causing inflammation and/or ulcerations. If left untreated, this inflammation can create more serious complications, such as narrowing of the intestinal passageways (**strictures**) that increase the risk of blockages, or **fistulas**, which are abnormal tunnels connecting the intestines and other adjacent structures, such as an abscess (collection of pus) near the anus called a perianal fistula. These conditions are relapsing and remitting, meaning that affected people will commonly experience flare-ups in which there is active inflammation in the affected area of the intestines, followed by periods of remission, in which there is little or no detectable inflammation or symptoms. However, there are people who may have no symptoms yet still have ongoing, undetected intestinal inflammation.

As is the case for other autoinflammatory diseases, the causes of IBD are not perfectly well understood. There is often an inherited component to it—IBD can run in families—but there is also likely an environmental trigger (or triggers) that can set it off in an already genetically predisposed person. For example, studies suggest that risk of developing IBD is higher for people who received multiple courses of antibiotics early in infancy/childhood compared with people who were exposed to fewer antibiotics. There are also studies that link our habitual diets in adolescence to risk of developing IBD later in life, with higher intake of fruits, vegetables, and/or fish during the teen years seeming to have a protective effect. Research findings of this nature strongly suggest that the health and diversity of our gut's inner ecosystem of bacteria and other microorganisms, collectively known as the gut microbiota, plays a role in the genesis of IBD. In fact, there are some studies that link the presence of a particular species of bacteria in the gut to risk of developing IBD. The microbiota, and which species may be increased or decreased in IBD, is being studied very intensively. So far, however, probiotics or antibiotics have not been found to be consistently helpful in managing IBD.

Inflammatory bowel diseases are conditions that we can't cure; the treatment goal is to quiet the immune system and send the disease into a hibernation of sorts—which medically is referred to as being in **remission**. While your doctor is working with you on identifying the right dose and combination of medications to help achieve remission, the role of diet is to help you manage symptoms of the still-active disease and ensure you are meeting your nutrition needs. The exception to this is for ulcerative colitis, which can essentially be permanently cured by a surgery called a **total proctocolectomy**, in which the entire colon is removed. Most people who undergo this surgery have a new rectum created by the surgeon in a series of operations, and this is referred to as an ileoanal anastomosis (or J pouch, since the new intestine is sewn in the shape of the letter J). For obvious reasons, this is not a first or even a second resort but is done when the disease is very severe, unresponsive to medications, and/or becomes complicated in a way that can cause dangerous side effects, like perforations of the bowel or when precancerous cells or cancer develops after many years of having colitis.

How Diarrhea from IBD Presents

Let's start by stating that not everyone with IBD experiences diarrhea. Some people have no changes in their bowel movements at all—their main complaint is abdominal pain—and some people, particularly those with Crohn's disease, even experience constipation! However, a change in bowel movements is an extremely common symptom for both Crohn's disease and ulcerative colitis, and diarrhea is more common than constipation, which is why I've chosen to place this chapter in the diarrhea section of the book.

Loose stools, frequent stools, urgent stools, and overt diarrhea are common among people with IBD. It is not uncommon to be awakened overnight with diarrhea or an urgent bowel movement, and there may also be blood and/or mucus in the stool. While some people have most of their bowel movements in the morning or earlier part of the day, others will feel the need to go soon after eating anything, and some will have to go regardless of whether they eat at all throughout the day. (In these latter cases, many of my patients with active IBD will minimize eating as much as they can early in the day so they can make it through work or school without provoking abdominal pain or urgent bowel movements. However, this often traps them in a vicious cycle of eating quite a bit at night, which then aggravates symptoms at bedtime, overnight, and/or the following morning.)

Often, diarrhea or bowel movements are accompanied by abdominal pain, though there may also be chronic abdominal pain even when you are not moving your bowels. Nausea and loss of appetite are a common complaint. People with Crohn's disease in particular can experience severe fatigue. With ulcerative colitis, fatigue may be a more direct result from iron-deficiency anemia, which is the main nutritional deficiency that can result from it, due primarily to loss of blood in the stool. In Crohn's, fatigue may or may not be associated with iron deficiency, and people are susceptible to nutritional deficiencies as well, which result not just from diarrheal losses but also impaired nutrient absorption from inflamed segments of the small intestine, or from self-imposed diet restrictions in an attempt to manage symptoms. These include (but are not limited to) vitamin B_6, vitamin B_{12}, folic acid, and minerals such as iron, zinc, copper, and selenium.

Diagnosing IBD

Stool tests

Often, the first step in diagnosing IBD involves a stool test that measures a marker of inflammation called **calprotectin**. If calprotectin levels in your stool sample are elevated beyond the normal range, you will likely require additional testing to identify where the inflammation seems to be occurring. If inflammation is in the colon—a condition called **colitis**—further evaluation is needed to determine whether it is colitis related to Crohn's disease, ulcerative colitis, or another type of colitis entirely. Believe it or not, these nuances matter quite a bit. The underlying nature of your colitis is going to determine what types of treatment it will best respond to. For example, colitis caused by specific, identifiable infections rather than IBD may respond to antibiotics or even over-the-counter medications such as Pepto-Bismol (bismuth subsalicylate), whereas colitis related to IBD often requires medications that work by targeting the immune system's overzealous behavior.

Endoscopy

If your stool calprotectin levels are elevated, your gastroenterologist will likely need to do some further testing to identify the nature of your inflammation, and this may take the form of a colonoscopy and/or upper endoscopy. Both colonoscopy and upper endoscopy involve the insertion of a long, flexible tube equipped with a video camera—called an endoscope—into your digestive tract. The endoscope is inserted into your well-prepped, empty colon via the anus (butthole) in the case of a colonoscopy. For an upper endoscopy, the scope goes in through your mouth, down your esophagus, through the stomach, and peeks into the first section of the small intestine. Both procedures are done under sedation. During the procedure(s), your doctor will likely obtain small tissue samples (biopsies) to send to a lab so that the tissue can be examined under a microscope for evidence of inflammation, though in the case of Crohn's disease and ulcerative colitis, inflammation will typically be visible to your doctor's naked eye through the scope.

Colonoscopy enables visual access to the entirety of your colon and usually to a small segment at the tail end of your small intestine, known as the **terminal ileum**, which means it is sufficient for diagnosing and monitoring ulcerative colitis, which only affects the colon. As described above, upper endoscopy enables visual access to the entirety of the esophagus, stomach, and the very beginning segment of your small intestine—a limited view when you need to diagnose something like Crohn's disease, which can affect any portion of the digestive tract, but in most cases these upper regions are not affected by Crohn's disease activity. For this reason, there are alternative forms of endoscopy that may be required to help your doctor visualize what's happening throughout the majority of the small intestine.

Capsule endoscopy involves swallowing a video-camera-equipped, onetime-use pill that usually obtains images of the entirety of the small intestine. The camera sends images of the digestive tract via radio signal to a recorder you wear for the duration of the test. The test lasts eight hours or until you poop out the video camera pill, whichever comes first. You do not need to stay in the doctor's office for the whole duration of the test, and you don't need to fish out and retrieve the capsule after pooping it out; your gastroenterologist uses a new one for the next person.

Blood Tests

Blood tests are done to check routine measurements such as your blood cell counts, measures of nutrition status, liver function, kidney function, electrolyte balance, and markers of inflammation—namely, C-reactive protein (CRP) and the erythrocyte sedimentation rate (ESR). They are not used to diagnose IBD per se.

Diagnostic Imaging

Diagnostic imaging is also available to help your doctor diagnose Crohn's disease—both its location and severity. A type of X-ray imaging called computed tomography (**CT scan**) is more helpful than traditional X-rays because it shows cross sections of your insides, provides three-dimensional pictures, and offers more details, especially of soft tissues and blood vessels. A type of CT scan called CT enterography (CTE) is better able to visualize the thickness of the bowel wall than even traditional CT scans, and is often used in the diagnosis or assessment of Crohn's disease. Another type of imaging called magnetic resonance enterography (MRE) is another option for aiding in the diagnosis and monitoring of Crohn's disease activity in the small intestine. Like CT scans, MRE offers a very detailed view of the small intestine, but unlike CT scans, it does not involve any radiation exposure.

Medical Treatment for IBD

There are many different types of medications used to manage IBD, each with its own set of benefits and risks. The choice of medication will be done in consultation with your doctor and may change over time. This section will offer a brief description of the various families of medications, though not all the medications will be appropriate for or offered to all people.

Corticosteroids

Corticosteroids are immune-system-suppressing medications that aim to tamp down the inappropriately overactive immune system in people with IBD, but their use is not limited to IBD. They may be given in pill form to be taken by mouth or via enemas delivered through the rectum. Examples include prednisone, methylprednisolone, and cortisone suppositories or foam. Another form of steroid that is not associated with the many steroid-induced side effects is budesonide, which is available as an oral pill or as a rectal foam preparation.

Aminosalicylates

Aminosalicylates (5-ASAs) are anti-inflammatory medications used for ulcerative colitis and are still used in Crohn's disease, particularly when the Crohn's activity is concentrated in the colon, but recent evidence does not demonstrate their effectiveness in people with Crohn's disease. Examples include mesalamine (Asacol, Pentasa, Lialda), sulfasalazine (Azulfidine), olsalazine (Dipentum), and balsalazide (Colazal). Rectal administration of 5-ASA medications can be accomplished via enemas (Rowasa) or suppositories (Canasa).

Immunomodulators

Immunomodulators are drugs that suppress the immune system and are often used as a second-line treatment when corticosteroids or 5-ASA medications have not been adequate. Certain immunomodulators are also used to treat other autoimmune diseases or even some forms of cancer. Examples include azathioprine (Imuran), 6-mercaptopurine (6-MP), and methotrexate.

Antibiotics

Antibiotics are medications that suppress bacterial populations in the gut; they're primarily used to treat infections. In Crohn's disease, antibiotics may be used to treat complications from the inflammation, such as perianal abscesses or fistulas. Antibiotics such as ciprofloxacin (Cipro) and metronidazole (Flagyl) have been used to treat Crohn's disease but have largely been replaced by more effective therapies.

Biologics

Biologics are lab-grown antibodies infused into the bloodstream directly via an intravenous infusion (infliximab [Remicade] or vedolizumab [Entyvio]), or by injection into the skin (adalimumab [Humira], ustekinumab [Stelara], golimumab [Simponi], certolizumab pegol [Cimzia]). These antibodies actively target certain proteins that are fueling inflammation. In the past, they had been given to people who have not responded adequately to the classes of medications described previously, but more and more, they may be tried even before immunomodulators. More recently, additional medications have been approved for people with moderate to severe inflammation, including tofacitinib (Xeljanz), ozanimod (Zeposia), and upadacitinib (Rinvoq).

Over-the-Counter Antidiarrheals

Over-the-counter antidiarrheals may also be used for people with ulcerative colitis to help with symptom management, though they do not help induce disease remission. Loperamide (Imodium) may be recommended by your doctor; it acts on local opioid receptors in the gut to slow down intestinal contractions that propel stool forward. This allows time for excess water in the bowel to be reabsorbed back into the body—helping to form stools—and should reduce the frequency of defecation as well. However, since loperamide does not readily cross the blood-brain barrier, it does not have the pain-killing effects that opioid narcotic painkillers do. Bismuth subsalicylate (Pepto-Bismol) may also control diarrhea by decreasing the flow of electrolytes and fluid into the bowel. These two medications can even be taken together.

Dietary Management of IBD

The primary goals of diet for IBD are twofold: to help reduce the severity of symptoms by choosing foods that do not aggravate your sensitive system, and to ensure your nutritional needs are being met when you may be malabsorbing some nutrients or avoiding certain foods or food groups because of tolerance issues. These are my immediate priorities as a dietitian when I work with patients who have IBD, and for good reason: Studies suggest that up to 30% of nonhospitalized patients with inflammatory bowel disease may be malnourished! Even when there is no obvious **malnutrition** in terms of inadequate intake of calories or protein, low body weight, or specific vitamin/mineral deficiencies, I still need to consider long-term nutritional consequences of my patients' medical treatments. For example, when my patients need to use steroid medications for long periods of time or are prone to repeated steroid treatments, I often need to make sure we're adequately supplementing calcium and vitamin D to protect bone mineral density. Like I said: IBD is a really complex disease to manage both medically and nutritionally.

But beyond these primary nutritional goals, there are some secondary nutritional goals to consider as well. When tolerance makes it possible, I do try to steer my patients toward anti-inflammatory dietary patterns that are increasingly associated with improved disease control and may support prolonged periods of remission. And believe it or not, one of the most anti-inflammatory compounds in the human diet is fiber.

Once upon a time, it was common practice for doctors and dietitians to recommend low-fiber diets to everyone with IBD. Chicken and rice, meat and potatoes, eggs and toast, Cream of Wheat cereal and Corn Flakes. No fruits other than bananas or applesauce. No veggies other than the occasional cooked carrot or cream of tomato soup.

We now know so much better. Research has shown that fiber is NOT your enemy when you have IBD. In fact, a growing body of evidence strongly points to the fact that including fiber in your diet when you have IBD is linked to better outcomes in terms of reduced number of flares and longer time in between flare-ups. For people with ulcerative colitis who have had a surgery to remove their entire colon (colectomy) and the creation of an intestinal pouch to help hold waste, higher-fiber diets are also associated with fewer instances of **pouchitis**—or an inflammation of the surgically created pouch. Because fiber feeds the gut microbiota, many of whose bacterial inhabitants produce anti-inflammatory compounds called short-chain fatty acids (SCFAs) as a result of fermenting this fiber, it makes sense that fiber intake can promote a less inflammatory environment in the gut. Feeding the gut microbes adequate fiber also helps ensure a thicker, intact mucous layer lining the gut. This mucous layer has an important barrier function that helps prevent bacteria from interacting with—and provoking—immune cells in the deeper layers of the bowel wall.

Fiber Intake for GI Tolerance

Nowadays, doctors and dietitians in the know are increasingly tailoring our fiber recommendations to each individual person, often manipulating the type and particle size of the fiber to help make it tolerable symptom-wise. Fiber tolerance will often vary based on whether you're in an active flare or in a remission, so it can be helpful to think of your diet as having a few different versions that you can transition between as needed.

As a general rule, a type of fiber called **soluble fiber** is more digestively tolerable than the roughage-type called **insoluble fiber**, and this is especially so when the food is going to be eaten whole or intact (as opposed to pureed). When it comes to soluble-fiber-predominant veggies, cooked is often better than raw. For example, cooked winter squash, zucchini, carrots, asparagus tips, and green beans are often the most tolerated veggies among my patients with both types of IBD, whereas skinless or seedless fruits like papaya, melon, avocado, banana, peeled pears, peeled/baked apples, and canned peaches are among the safest choices in that category. Oats are typically the best tolerated whole-grain food, especially in somewhat more refined textures, like instant oatmeal, Cheerios, or oat flour–based crackers. See Chapter 12, page 244, for a more comprehensive list of soluble-fiber-predominant foods.

Plenty of people with IBD can tolerate fiber-containing foods beyond this small core of relatively safer soluble fiber options when they take measures to reduce the particle size of the fiber—whichever type of fiber it is—from its whole, intact form to a more refined or even pureed form. Picture the physical properties of insoluble fiber–rich chopped, raw kale tossed together in a salad bowl; it's coarse, it's bulky, and as mouthful after mouthful of chewed-up leaves start passing through an inflamed segment of the intestine, you could imagine how it would almost have a scrub brush-like effect on the already raw and angry tissue. But picture the physical properties of a green smoothie made with that same bowl of raw kale leaves; having been blenderized into a smooth, silky liquid, it could glide right over that inflamed segment of the bowel wall without aggravating things much, if at all. By manipulating the physical, textural properties of higher-fiber foods, many people with IBD find that they can comfortably consume a more nutrient-rich, varied, fiber-containing diet that helps in the fight against inflammation through its positive impact on the gut microbiota.

Reducing the particle size of fiber can be helpful when you are in a flare, and is also an essential safety practice for people with Crohn's disease who have a history of small bowel obstructions due to strictures or scar tissue even when in remission. Bulky, intact fiber can become logjammed at narrowed segments of the bowel and create blockages that represent a medical emergency and may even require surgery to resolve. However, as I like to tell my patients who are living with adhesions, scar tissue, and strictures: "If it can fit through a straw, it can fit through your strictured bowel!" Besides, soup is basically like liquid salad—it has all the same vitamins and nutrients as raw, intact veggies, just in a different, gentler form. If

Table 7-1: Plant-Based Foods with
Small-Particle-Size Fiber for Tolerance

Fruits	Applesauce
	Banana
	Guacamole or mashed avocado
	Kids' pureed fruit/veggie squeeze pouches (don't knock them till you try them!)
	Smoothies (berries and any/all fruits or leafy greens OK, as long as they are well pureed)
Veggies	Butternut squash soufflé
	Canned crushed tomatoes; marinara/tomato sauce; romesco sauce
	Gazpacho
	Green juices
	Mashed cauliflower (like mashed potatoes)
	Mashed sweet potato (no skins)
	Pesto sauce (well-blended version, not too chunky)
	Pureed vegetable soups (asparagus, borscht, broccoli, carrot ginger, cauliflower, pumpkin, tomato,)
	Roasted red pepper sauce
	Tomato juice or V-8
	Thanksgiving-style root vegetable puree (carrots, parsnips, sweet potato, turnips)
Plant-based proteins	Fully pureed bean or lentil soups
	Hemp hearts
	Hummus
	Pumfu ("tofu" made from pumpkin seeds)
	Smooth refried beans
	Tofu

(continues)

Table 7-1 *(continued)*

Nuts/seeds	Cashew-based vegan cheeses
	Nondairy nut "milks" (Elmhurst 1925 brand makes them with more actual nut nutrition and no added thickeners)
	Nut butters (almond, cashew, peanut)
	Seed butters (pumpkin seed butter, sunflower seed butter, tahini)
	Vegan cashew "cream" sauce
Whole grains	Bob's Red Mill Creamy Brown Rice cereal (cooked cereal)
	Bob's Red Mill Creamy Buckwheat cereal (cooked cereal)
	Cheerios
	Instant oatmeal
	Oatmilk
	Quinoa flakes (cooked cereal)

you are at risk for bowel obstructions, invest in a high-powered blender or food processor, and populate your diet with smoothies and pureed soups, which are small-particle-size versions of healthy plant-based foods.

Managing Overall Diet for GI Tolerance

Other factors that affect diet tolerance in IBD—especially when you're in a flare—include:

- **Meal size/portions:** Eating less volume at a time will be less stimulating to the bowel's normal reflexes and may help reduce cramping, pain, and/or diarrhea. Smaller food volume consumed at once also reduces the likelihood of obstructing the bowel if you have a stricture.

- **Fat:** Digestion of higher-fat meals creates the bowel-stimulating nerve reflex called the gastrocolic reflex, which I first described in Chapter 2. If you recall, this digestive nerve signal can activate cramping, pain, or urgent bowel movements in sensitive individuals. Avoiding fatty foods like fattier cuts of red meat, fried foods, cream sauces, cheese sauces, ice cream, oily/greasy takeout food, and similarly high-fat choices is often helpful during a flare.

- **"Osmotic" sugars:** Natural sugars like lactose (milk sugar), sorbitol, and/or fructose can draw extra water into the bowel and aggravate diarrhea. Lactose-free dairy foods are often better tolerated—especially during a flare. Concentrated sources of fructose or sorbitol—like from larger servings of juices, soft drinks/soda, dried fruit, or certain summer fruits like cherries or watermelon—may also aggravate diarrhea. See Chapter 13 for lists of foods high in these osmotic sugars that may be problematic, especially in larger portions.

Addressing Malnutrition and Nutritional Deficiencies

In cases where you struggle to maintain a healthy body weight or get in enough protein, your doctor or dietitian may recommend you include some liquid meal supplements in your regular diet to bridge nutritional gaps. This can be especially helpful when your appetite is poor or when you are having a hard time tolerating solid food. Products like Ensure (Abbott Nutrition) and Boost (Nestlé Health Science) are well-known and widely available, and both companies also market a clear, juice-like, fat-free version of their product (Ensure Clear and Boost Breeze, respectively) when the fat/creaminess of the original products seem problematic. More recently, companies have been responding to consumer demand for more natural, real-food-based liquid meal replacement products, or at least products that do not contain as many (or any) food additives. Examples of these include Ensure Harvest and PediaSure Harvest (Abbott Nutrition), Compleat (Nestlé Health Science), Nourish and Liquid Hope (Functional Formularies), and Real Food Blends (Nutricia).

Anti-Inflammatory Diet Patterns
to Support Remission

Inflammatory bowel diseases are perhaps the most extensively studied of all digestive conditions, which is why it never fails to surprise
me that there is relatively little research into the role of diet as a
supporting pillar of a thorough treatment plan. When I first started
practicing over a decade ago, patients would come to me seeking
nutrition advice on both managing their IBD symptoms as well
as eating to help promote healing. Commonly, they'd report that
their doctors dismissed their interest in nutrition as irrelevant to the
treatment plan, advising them that "it doesn't matter what you eat,"
and that IBD can only be treated with drugs.

Exclusive Enteral Nutrition

With emerging (but still far too limited) research, we know now
that this isn't entirely true. There still isn't great evidence that diet
alone can send IBD into remission or that therapeutic diets can take
the place of medication. The most promising evidence of diet as an
actual treatment for IBD involves complete liquid diets for six to
twelve weeks as part of a regimen called **exclusive enteral nutrition (EEN)**. EEN, which involves avoiding all solid foods and living off nutritionally complete, commercially available liquid meal
replacements like Ensure, Boost, or their medical food equivalents
typically used in hospitals (or see list of natural alternatives in the
previous section), has been better studied as a solo treatment option
for children than it has been for adults. For example, EEN has been
shown to be slightly more effective than steroid treatments in inducing remission in children with Crohn's disease. In adults, the modest amount of available research suggests that medications appear to
be more effective than EEN in inducing remission as a solo therapy,
though there is some suggestion from a 2017 study that a period of
EEN before surgery may reduce the need to even have surgery or
reduce postoperative complications among those who still require

it. If you are considering EEN as a treatment option, it is essential to discuss the potential risks of delaying medication treatment with your doctor, which will be based on the severity of your disease. You should also meet with a registered dietitian who has experience guiding other patients through these protocols; they will help you identify a tolerable product that meets your needs and that you find palatable enough to live off for two to three months; advise how much of the formula you will need to drink daily to meet your complete nutritional needs; and help make sure you can get your insurance company to reimburse the expense.

Partial Enteral Nutrition

If drinking nothing but meal replacement shakes for two to three months feels like a way greater commitment than you have the emotional reserve to undertake, research is underway regarding **partial enteral nutrition (PEN),** in which you replace some—but not all—of your solid meals with liquid meal replacements. A study published in 2015 combined data from a bunch of smaller studies of patients with moderate to severe Crohn's disease who were taking the medication infliximab (Remicade) and found that people who combined the medication with a diet protocol in which they adhered to PEN were twice as likely to achieve disease remission compared with those who were only taking the medication without PEN, and close to three times more likely to remain in remission a year later. The effective regimen of PEN involved participants getting at least 600 of their daily calories from liquid formulas instead of solid food, and most (but not all) of these formulas were elemental formulas in which the nutrients were broken down by enzymes to be quickly and easily digestible. More research is needed, however, to offer more precise guidelines for those of us in clinical practice so we can offer individualized advice to our patients. In the absence of this research, however, it would not be unreasonable for well-nourished patients to work with a dietitian on replacing one or two of your three meals (or a meal and a snack) per day with a nutritionally balanced liquid meal for a period of time, especially if the solid meal(s) you eat are part of one of the anti-inflammatory diet patterns described later in this chapter.

As the above study on PEN demonstrates, while there isn't yet a strong case to be made for diet alone being able to induce remission in IBD on its own for most adults, there is far more compelling evidence that points to diet functioning in a "best supporting actor" role, essentially enhancing the effectiveness of medical treatments; helping to speed up the achievement of remission compared with just taking medicine alone; and helping patients who are in remission reduce the likelihood of a flare-up. It's been quite some time since I've heard of a doctor telling their patients with IBD that diet doesn't matter at all, as there is increasing recognition in the medical community that our food choices affect the gut microbiota, and in turn, the gut microbiota interact with our immune system in a way that can influence inflammation.

The International Organization for the Study of Inflammatory Bowel Disease (IOIBD) has issued diet recommendations based on the best available research we have about the connection between eating patterns and IBD disease risk and outcomes. They offer some general guidelines about ingredients and foods to avoid, as well as some specific guidelines for foods to emphasize and eat more of, depending on what type of IBD you have.

According to 2020 guidelines published by the IOIBD, it is prudent for people with IBD to try *minimizing their intake* of ultra-processed foods that contain specific additives that have been associated with disruptions in the gut's barrier function or that affect the microbiota in an unfavorable way. See the sidebar for a list of the foods and ingredients in question.

FOODS AND INGREDIENTS
TO LIMIT WHEN YOU HAVE IBD

Ingredients in packaged foods and beverages:

- Carrageenan

- Maltodextrin

- Titanium dioxide

- Artificial sweeteners

- Certain emulsifers, such as mono- and diglycerides, poly-sorbates, carboxymethylcellulose

Foods high in saturated fat, including:

- Red meat (beef, lamb, pork)

- Dairy fat (butter, cream, cheese, whole milk)

- Coconut oil

- Palm oil

- Processed meats, such as bacon, hot dogs, ham, salami, cold cuts

Source: Adapted from the International Organization for Inflammatory Bowel Disease (IOIBD)

Evidence linking frequent intake of ultra-processed foods and risk of developing IBD continues to mount. In 2021, the *British Journal of Medicine* published a very large study that tracked the dietary habits and health outcomes of 116,000 people over a nine-year period. In this study, the tally of ultra-processed foods included a variety of items, including soft drinks; salty snacks like chips; sweet treats like packaged cookies, cakes, and bars; and processed meats. The researchers found that the more servings of ultra-processed foods a person consumed in a day, the greater was their risk of developing IBD over the course of the study, and that the risk increased in a dose-dependent way. Specifically, compared with people who consumed less than one serving of these foods per day (on average), people who consumed five or more servings per day had an 82% greater risk of developing IBD. The risk was 67% greater for people who consumed one to four servings per day.

On the flip side, there are certain foods that may be protective and beneficial that people with IBD may consider trying to eat more of. People with ulcerative colitis are encouraged to consume more fish, seafood, and other foods rich in omega-3 fats, which have an anti-inflammatory effect. Beyond fish and seafood—for which fatty fish like salmon, herring, and mackerel are the best sources—other omega-3-rich foods include walnuts, flaxseeds (whole or ground), flaxseed oil, chia seeds, and hemp hearts (shelled hemp seeds); many of these can be added to other foods like oatmeal, smoothies, or yogurt to ensure you get at least one good portion in each day. For Crohn's disease, available data suggests that high intake of fruits and vegetables may be beneficial.

As I mentioned earlier in the chapter, such fiber-forward recommendations sometimes surprise my patients, who are often under the impression that the recommended diet for IBD is a low-fiber one. But while it's true that it's been common practice for decades to advise low-fiber diets in IBD—largely due to the reality that many IBD patients do not tolerate very fibrous foods like salad or nuts—we now have a more nuanced understanding of the role of fiber in IBD. Because medically speaking, fiber seems to be more of a friend than a foe, the issue in practice is to figure out how we can manipulate the physical texture of fiber to make it gentler and facilitate digestive tolerance rather than having people avoid fiber altogether.

Two of the more commonly used diets to manage IBD symptoms that spotlight fiber from fruits and veggies and limit highly processed foods as per the IOIBD recommendations are the specific carbohydrate diet (SCD) and the Mediterranean diet. As of the time of this writing, there is only a modest amount of research into the benefits of these respective dietary patterns for people with IBD. From what we know so far, both seem promising in terms of their potential to improve symptoms and reduce inflammatory markers, and neither one appears measurably superior to the other.

Specific Carbohydrate Diet

The **specific carbohydrate diet** (SCD) is a grain-free, low-sugar, low-dairy diet that was popularized in the 1990s by a book called *Breaking the Vicious Cycle*, written by a biochemist named Elaine Gottschall whose child had great success in managing their ulcerative colitis on the diet. Gottschall based the book on the work of pediatrician Sidney Haas, who devised the diet in the World War II era initially as a treatment for celiac disease. The diet became popular within the IBD community largely through word of mouth, as the book was published just prior to the internet age. Its popularity was fueled by testimonials of patients who reported significant improvements in their symptoms and disease severity upon adopting the diet. However, it took several decades for researchers to seek funding to test this diet in a controlled way to provide some non-anecdotal evidence about whether the diet could actually be expected to improve symptoms, reduce inflammation, promote remission—or any combination of these outcomes—compared with control diets.

A SAMPLE GENTLE-TEXTURED MENU ON THE SPECIFIC CARBOHYDRATE DIET

Breakfast
Omelet with spinach, tomato, and Swiss cheese and a side of cut melon

+ Black coffee

Lunch
Homemade lentil vegetable soup (pureed as needed for tolerance) with a side of homemade almond flour crackers dipped in homemade guacamole

Snack
Peeled apple slices or banana with natural/no-sugar-added cashew butter

Dinner
Baked/grilled salmon or chicken served with mashed cauliflower and cooked string beans with olive oil and salt

---

The SCD is a whole foods–based diet; essentially everything you eat will be homemade from minimally processed ingredients. It prohibits all grains and starchy root vegetables, including starches like sweet potatoes and/or tapioca flour that are allowed on more popular grain-free diets, like Paleo or Whole30. Chickpeas and soybeans are prohibited, but certain other legumes, like lentils, are allowed. Nuts are allowed but seeds are not. The only sugar allowed is from honey (in small amounts), fresh fruit, freshly squeezed fruit juices, and dried fruits. The only dairy allowed is lactose-free; this includes butter, hard/aged cheese, and plain yogurt that you make yourself at home. (Commercial lactose-free milk, however, is prohibited.) Processed meats are also prohibited, including cold cuts, hot dogs, and sausages. Of note—and much to my chagrin—Gottschall and her disciples refer to included foods as "SCD legal" and excluded foods as "SCD illegal." I worry that thinking about foods this way can really do a number on a person's relationship with food—as if having IBD doesn't already cause a fraught relationship with food and eating on its own. I think that even if you choose to follow the SCD, it's important to bear in mind that some "SCD illegal" foods—like whole grains, potatoes, chickpeas, and soybeans—are allowed and even encouraged on the Mediterranean diet, which has thus far shown itself to be equally beneficial for patients with mild to moderate Crohn's disease. In other words, it is reasonable to hypothesize that the SCD's apparent helpfulness may have more to do with its emphasis on high-fiber intake and avoidance of highly processed foods rather than on its exclusion of all grains and starches. This is where more research would really come in handy.

As you can see based on this set of restrictions, the foundations of a specific carbohydrate diet are animal proteins (eggs, fish, chicken, meat), nuts or minimally processed nut butters, cheese, fruits, fresh non-starchy vegetables (canned foods are discouraged), and some beans/legumes—like lentils, black beans, and kidney beans—ideally cooked from dry rather than canned. With the extensive list of restrictions, you may be happy to learn that the occasional vodka is allowed, as are freshly squeezed fruit juice mixers. See the side bar on page 154 for a sample day's menu on the SCD; I featured this softer-textured version featuring cooked veggies, skinless fruits, and some more pureed options that may be gentler and easier to tolerate than a version that features raw veggies/salads, whole nuts, and other intact forms of "roughage" that many people with IBD can find hard to tolerate. See Chapter 12 for a lengthier discussion on this approach to fiber modification.

Because the SCD is a lower-carb diet, some people find that they lose weight. If you cannot maintain a healthy body weight on the SCD, then it is NOT the right diet for you, as the risks of developing malnutrition in the setting of autoimmune disease outweigh the potential benefits of this diet. A less restrictive, Mediterranean diet may be a better fit for you. Similarly, if you don't cook or can't cook, the SCD is also not the right diet for you. This diet prohibits use of practically any packaged convenience foods, and it all but eliminates your ability to eat out or order in from restaurants. To follow the SCD, you must be willing and able to devote significant time to cooking foods from scratch and packing your own meals/ snacks to take with you on the road.

Mediterranean Diet

The **Mediterranean diet**, which I will henceforth refer to as the "Med diet" (to avoid having to keep typing out and inevitably misspelling "Mediterranean") gets a lot of great press for very good reasons. It's a dietary pattern that, as of the time of this writing, has thus far been strongly associated with reduced risk of developing cardiovascular disease, type 2 diabetes, breast cancer, colorectal cancer, inflammatory bowel disease, Alzheimer's disease and cognitive decline, nonalcoholic fatty liver disease, and frailty in old age. By the time this book winds up in your hands, the list will probably even be longer.

A SAMPLE GENTLE-TEXTURED MENU ON THE MEDITERRANEAN DIET

Breakfast
Oatmeal served with cinnamon, almond butter, blueberries, or peeled/diced pear

+ Coffee with a splash of low-fat milk

Lunch
Toasted Ezekiel bread or bakery sourdough bread with Italian tuna salad (made with olive oil, not mayo), avocado, and sliced tomatoes

+ Side of fresh sliced nectarines or peaches

Snack(s)
Hummus + soft veggie dippers (jarred roasted red pepper, steamed baby carrots, peeled/seeded cucumber spears, well-steamed cauliflower florets)

0% plain Greek yogurt sweetened with a drizzle of honey

Dinner
Pasta with white beans, pesto, and roasted zucchini (with or without shrimp or a small amount of chicken)

Dessert
A few squares of dark chocolate

The Med diet is a high-fiber diet whose foundation is plant-based foods like whole grains, beans, vegetables, fruits, and nuts; all these foods are meant to be consumed daily in some form or another. It also emphasizes high intake of heart-healthy, anti-inflammatory unsaturated fats from olive oil, and also fish and nuts. It is not necessarily a dairy-free diet, but dairy is not a daily staple on the diet and is used sparingly—think low-fat Greek yogurt or a feta sprinkle on a salad or some cooked veggies. Red meat is consumed very seldom, if at all, certainly no more than a small portion once or twice per month. Because of the minimal inclusion of dairy and red meat, the Med diet is very low in saturated fats, which are known to be more pro-inflammatory. Incidentally, coconut oil is also very high in saturated fat and would be discouraged on any science-based, anti-inflammatory diet pattern. Don't let the online wellness community's health-washing campaign convince you that coconut oil is somehow a healthy fat or that it has anti-inflammatory powers.

As you will see, the Med diet differs from the SCD in that it not only allows but actually encourages whole grains and beans/legumes as daily staples; it also emphasizes relatively high intake of olive oil and unsaturated fats, whereas the SCD is somewhat agnostic about the type and amount of fat intake. Both diets are rather low in dairy but not necessarily strictly dairy-free, and both diets eschew highly processed foods in favor of whole, minimally processed ones, though convenient staples like canned tomatoes, canned tuna, or canned beans would certainly be allowed on a Med diet as the sample diet in the sidebar suggests.

The first randomized controlled study that attempted to compare these diets head-to-head as therapeutic interventions for people with IBD—in this case, for people with mild to moderate Crohn's disease—was published in 2021 in the journal *Gastroenterology*. The study lasted for twelve weeks and included close to two hundred participants who did not have known strictures (narrowing of the bowels) or a history of bowel obstructions. They were allowed to remain on their usual regimen of Crohn's medications; this means that the study was really investigating diet as an adjunctive (add-on) therapy to medication, not as a primary treatment itself. Participants in both the SCD group and the Med diet group achieved symptom remission within six weeks at comparable rates (43% vs. 46%), and a smaller but similar percentage of people on each diet (31% vs. 35%) also experienced substantial reductions in fecal calprotectin levels, which is a marker for severity of inflammation in IBD. The authors concluded that neither diet was superior than the other in terms of therapeutic benefit, and the diet that one finds easier to follow would probably be the better choice. (In this case, the authors took a position that the Med diet may be preferable given its relatively lower level of restrictiveness, and also because of the other health benefits it is known to have.)

A key point to note about this study is that it is the first one I've seen that offers some ballpark idea about what percentage of people can expect to derive a benefit from one of the better-studied anti-inflammatory diet patterns for IBD. As the above numbers suggest, just under half of people with similar disease characteristics as those in the study who adopt an SCD or Med diet might expect substantial improvement in symptoms, and about one-third of them might expect improvement in underlying inflammation within six weeks. In other words, one of these diets may not be an effective add-on treatment for everyone, but it seems extremely helpful for a substantial-enough percentage of people that it is worth a try!

Unfortunately, we don't yet have much data to tell us what diet(s) may be best for people with ulcerative colitis and what percentage of people with UC can expect results from diet change and whether it is comparable to the rates observed to date among people with Crohn's.

Dietary Supplements for IBD

The primary role of dietary supplements is to correct deficiencies or prevent nutrition-related side effects of medications. Iron deficiency is extremely common among people with ulcerative colitis (due to losses of blood in the stool), and quite prevalent in Crohn's disease as well (due to the combined effect of malabsorption and blood losses). Iron supplements taken by mouth are the first-line treatment to correct iron deficiencies, though there can be tolerance issues—especially with higher-dose products. Some people find that splitting the dose into two or three moderate (18 mg to 28 mg) or even lower-dose supplements sits better in their system than taking a single high-dose supplement, which typically comes in 65 mg doses. For example, many children's chewable multivitamins with iron contain 18 mg per tablet (e.g., Flintstones with Iron) and may be tolerated relatively well if taken with food twice or three times daily to meet the dose recommended by your doctor. A product called Feosol Bifera contains 28 mg of a highly absorbable form of iron, and one to two per day may go a long way toward correcting less severe iron deficiencies. If you are looking to avoid some of the filler ingredients red-flagged by the IOIBD and listed earlier in this chapter, you can try Pure Encapsulations Iron-C (15 mg per pill), Solgar Chelated Iron (25 mg per pill), or Floradix Iron + Herbs (liquid, 10 mg per serving; contains gluten ingredients). Taking an immediate-release vitamin C supplement (chewable, gummy, powder, or liquid) may improve the absorption of the oral iron supplement.

Certain medications used to treat IBD—particularly those in the corticosteroid class—can have a negative effect on bone density. Examples of medications in this category are listed on page 140. If you will need to take steroids for any significant period of time, or find yourself hopping on and off courses of steroids over the course of your illness, it is prudent to supplement both calcium and vitamin D to help protect your bones and prevent medication-induced osteoporosis. The recommended dose of calcium for IBD patients with frequent corticosteroid use is 1,500 mg of calcium daily, and 1,000 IU of vitamin D, though higher doses of vitamin D may be recommended to you based on your personal blood levels. Similarly, if you choose to avoid or limit dairy for reasons of digestive tolerance or one of the therapeutic diets described above, talk to your doctor or dietitian about whether supplementing calcium and vitamin D make sense for you regardless of what medication regimen you follow. If you supplement calcium and iron, you should not take them at the same time, as they compete for absorption.

Other specific dietary supplements may be advised by your doctor or dietitian based on your individual circumstances. If you are losing a lot of weight because you are having difficulty eating enough, you may require a multivitamin or multi-mineral to help bridge gaps that you are missing from your diet. In other cases, specific deficiencies in vitamin B_6, vitamin B_{12}, folic acid, zinc, copper, selenium, or vitamin D may be detected and need to be corrected.

Beyond the role of supplements to correct specific nutritional deficiencies, many of my IBD patients are interested in whether certain supplements can have a therapeutic benefit on their disease itself. Often before a patient even lands in my office, they've been experimenting with a range of supplements or entire "gut-healing" protocols that are popular among online wellness influencers, naturopaths, and practitioners in the functional/integrative medicine and nutrition world. Supplements common to these protocols typically involve some cocktail of L-glutamine, probiotics, prebiotics derived from plant fiber or those structurally identical to molecules found in breast milk (human milk oligosaccharides), licorice root extract, slippery elm, and/or marshmallow root. Some companies market supplements that contain immune cells called immunoglobulins derived from the blood of cows, claiming that they support a healthy mucous barrier or bind toxic by-products of gut bacteria that can penetrate the gut's mucus barrier and activate immune cells.

In reality, there are only a small number of dietary supplements that have actually been tested in patients with IBD and emerged with some semblance of scientific evidence to support their use, and they apply more to people with ulcerative colitis than to those with Crohn's disease. They are listed below.

Curcumin

Curcumin is one of the active compounds in the culinary and medicinal herb we know as turmeric, which is responsible for the orangey-yellow color in foods common in the many cuisines that use it—particularly South Asian. It has a known anti-inflammatory effect. Available research from several small studies suggests that when a therapeutic dose of supplemental curcumin is added to standard medication regimens for mild to moderate ulcerative colitis (e.g., mesalamine), the odds of achieving remission are substantially improved when compared with using just the medication alone. In 2020, multiple review studies in which researchers pooled the results from several smaller studies found that adding curcumin to medical treatment increased the likelihood of achieving remission by anywhere from three to five times! Tolerance of the supplement is often reported to be very good, though as with all dietary supplements, there is always the possibility of adverse effects. Unfortunately, the dose of curcumin used in these smaller investigative studies varies quite a bit—from 450 mg on the low end to 3,000 mg (3 g) on the higher end—so it's hard to offer precise guidance about the therapeutic dose sweet spot. In my clinical practice, I've typically recommended 2,000 to 3,000 mg/d (2–3 g) in split doses.

If you are purchasing a turmeric or curcumin supplement, you may need to read labels carefully and do some math to make sure you are getting a therapeutic dose somewhere in the (wide) range described above. Supplement companies may label their products as having 1,000 mg of turmeric, but when you read the fine print in the "Supplement Facts" table, it discloses that their turmeric powder or extract only consists of, say, 35% curcuminoids. This means that the dose contains only 350 mg of actual curcumin—which may be too low to have a benefit. To figure out how much curcumin your supplement actually contains, you need to take the milligrams of total turmeric extract listed on the label per dose (500 mg, 1,200 mg, 1,600 mg, etc.) and multiply that by the percentage of curcuminoids claimed (.35 for 35%, .95 for 95%, etc.). The number you get tells you how many milligrams of curcumin you're actually getting per listed dose, which may be more than one pill.

Mixed/Eight-Strain Probiotics (Visbiome/VSL #3)

A high-potency cocktail of eight specific freeze-dried probiotic strains marketed under the brand Visbiome has been tested in randomized controlled trials in people with ulcerative colitis. Of note, most of the research into this cocktail was conducted using an earlier version of a product called VSL #3, which is still on the market but was reformulated in 2016 because of a rift between the researcher who developed the formulation and the company marketing it. (Probiotic politics can be ugly.) Visbiome's product is identical to the pre-2016 formulation of VSL #3 on which most of the available research is based. It is unclear whether the post-2016 modifications to the formulation of the product currently marketed as VSL #3 affect its efficacy relative to the prior formulation.

The strongest data support the use of this eight-strain probiotic cocktail to treat and prevent pouchitis in people who have undergone a colectomy surgery. In fact, evidence-based clinical guidelines on probiotic use issued by the American Gastroenterological Association (AGA) in 2020 concluded that there is only strong enough evidence to justify the use of these mixed probiotics for the treatment and prevention of pouchitis, not of ulcerative colitis itself.

Nonetheless, there are still some data suggesting that these eight-strain probiotics could be of benefit for people with mild to moderate ulcerative colitis who have not undergone surgery—whether alone (induction therapy) or when paired with medication (adjunctive therapy). A 2020 systematic review and meta-analysis of multiple smaller studies published in *PLOS One* found that compared with a placebo, old formula VSL #3/current Visbiome formula was about 2.4 times more likely to induce a clinical remission in people when used as a first-line treatment for people who were not taking any other medication.

There are only two small studies from the early 2000s that suggest a benefit of (old formulation) VSL #3—and ostensibly, current Visbiome—on increasing the odds of achieving remission when added to medications like 5-ASAs or immunomodulators compared with taking the medications alone, but the results were nonetheless promising. Because these probiotic products can be extremely expensive, it's hard to justify recommending them as a matter of course to anyone and everyone as an adjunctive therapy. However, if cost is not an issue for you, it would not be unreasonable to try adding one of these eight-strain probiotics to your medication regimen given their strong safety profile.

Case Study: Is It Crohn's or Is It SIBO?

Leah was a woman in her twenties who had been diagnosed with Crohn's disease affecting the second segment of her small intestine (jejunum) about six months prior. When I met her, she was already several months into taking a biologic medication called Humira. Prior to starting this medication, she'd have bad diarrhea, many times daily, and was also vomiting frequently. Now, her bowel patterns were all over the place and she was even having bouts of constipation. Some days she'd have urgency, but when she went to sit on the toilet, nothing came out, or there would be tiny little pellets she had to strain to get out. Other days, she'd eat something higher in fat and have terrible diarrhea. Most days, stools were pretty loose and she would go three times on average.

The Humira resolved her vomiting, but Leah was still struggling with terrible nausea, bloating, and a poor appetite. She couldn't stomach eating anything in the mornings, and when she did muster the ability to put something in her mouth, she wasn't craving foods that were particularly healthy. Rather—she would grab whatever was convenient, easy, and plain. Bagels, cookies, sandwiches with fries, candy. Because of the nausea, Leah sometimes went eighteen hours without eating a thing, and she had lost a significant amount of weight—over thirty pounds. It worried her that her diet lacked nutritional balance and she was eating so much "junk food," since she was someone who used to love cooking and eating vegetables prior to her Crohn's disease diagnosis. But who wants to eat salads when you're super-nauseated and your bowels are in constant tur- moil? Leah's relationship with eating was worsening by the week— food felt like the enemy—and it was taking a toll on her mental health as well as her physical health.

Her doctor assumed that these persistent symptoms were attrib- utable to the Crohn's disease and decided to increase her dose of Humira to see if it would help. Diet-wise, I suggested a variety of ways to increase the nutritional balance of Leah's diet in ways that wouldn't aggravate her nausea and might be easier to eat—ice-cold fruit smoothies sipped gradually in the morning, comforting veggie soups like pumpkin or carrot ginger, or mashed avocado toast with eggs. I also wondered whether going too long without eating could also be aggravating her nausea. While Leah did make some prog- ress in terms of introducing some more nutritious, gentle-textured fruits and vegetables into her diet and breaking up those long gaps between meals, she certainly didn't feel much better physically. Even after two months on a higher dose of her Humira, things still weren't improving measurably in terms of how she felt.

About three months after I first met with Leah, I finally sug- gested that perhaps we were missing something by focusing on her Crohn's disease as the only possible cause for all her symptoms. What if she had developed a concurrent case of small intestinal bac- terial overgrowth, or SIBO (see Chapter 6) as a result of small bowel inflammation from her Crohn's? Could that be responsible for some of her persistent problems? I suggested we have her undergo a breath test to investigate this possibility, but her doctor decided to just skip the test and prescribe an antibiotic called Xifaxan, which is commonly used to treat SIBO.

A month after the medication was prescribed, Leah was back on my schedule. She was all smiles. Her tone and her energy had shifted, and she looked vibrant and well. She'd been feeling "GREAT" since completing her antibiotic course, she told me. Her digestive symptoms were almost completely gone, and feeling physically good had naturally motivated her to want to reach for healthy foods more often. She was eating every few hours throughout the day, and was even tolerating things like spicy foods and some higher-fat foods that used to cause abdominal cramping or diarrhea. Her weight was starting to rebound back to a healthier level. She was even starting to exercise a bit. At this point, we both realized that it was almost certainly SIBO that had been dogging her all those months, and her Crohn's disease actually seemed to be under rather good control once the SIBO smoke screen had been removed.

Moving forward, Leah planned to continue focusing on a nutritious, fiber-forward diet rich in fruits and vegetables both because it felt much more realistic to do so now and because she knew that a diet richer in these foods and less reliant on heavily processed, less nutritious foods was one thing she could do to help promote an anti-inflammatory environment in her gut and keep her Crohn's disease quiet.

The Swollen Bowel

Histamine Intolerance

ONE OF THE LESSER-KNOWN CAUSES of acute diarrheal attacks is swelling in the bowels caused by high levels of histamine—a signaling compound that produces inflammatory reactions, typically in response to allergens or injuries.

Histamine is a molecule produced by certain types of white blood cells called mast cells and basophils. Its job is to rush to the site of an injury or sound the alarm when a foreign food or environmental protein invades the body. When it arrives on location, it enables our blood vessels to become leaky enough so they can deliver fluids full of the necessary compounds for healing to the site of an assault. It's this leakiness that produces swelling in response to insults as minor as mosquito bites and injuries as major as scrapes and wounds. Histamine is one of the chemical mediators involved in an immediate allergic reaction. White blood cells release it when they're signaled to do so by a type of antibody, called an IgE antibody, that recognizes a foreign food protein or environmental allergen (think pollen or dust mites) as having infiltrated the body. In extreme cases, this allergic reaction can be life-threatening; it may cause such severe swelling of the respiratory tract that the airways constrict and breathing is impeded, or a severe and dangerous drop in blood pressure. This type of reaction is called **anaphylaxis**. When histamine floods the gut, it can produce a swelling-type reaction that may result in sudden bloating, belly pain, vomiting, and/or watery diarrhea; it also provokes the release of stomach acid and may produce symptoms of acid reflux, heartburn, or indigestion.

Histamine is found naturally outside the human body as well. It's a natural by-product of bacterial breakdown of protein foods that contain a building block (amino acid) called histidine. This process of bacterial breakdown can occur deliberately through food preservation methods like culturing and curing, or unintentionally through spoilage. For example, histamine is produced when milk is cultured into yogurt or cheese, when steaks are dry aged, when meats are cured to become hard salamis, or when fish hangs around too long and starts to spoil. Elsewhere in nature, some foods just happen to be naturally high in histamine: the best available data suggest that tomatoes, spinach, eggplant, avocados, and yeast extracts are among them—though the best available data on histamine content of foods is admittedly not so great.

Histamine Intolerance

Histamine intolerance is an emerging diagnosis that describes an adverse reaction to consuming foods that are either high in preformed histamine or trigger the release of histamine by your own white blood cells. The reaction can take many forms and may cause symptoms in your digestive system, skin, circulatory system, or respiratory system. Histamine intolerance is thought to have its roots in the gut, presumably due to deficiency of an enzyme required to break down histamine in the digestive tract called **diamine oxidase (DAO)**. A DAO deficiency would mean that it takes the body longer to degrade a histamine load that arrives in the gut from food or that is produced in the gut by the resident bacteria, allowing this inflammatory compound to build up and wreak some havoc as it waits around to be broken down.

While it is possible to measure DAO enzyme levels in the blood, as of the time of this writing in late 2022, there is no solid evidence that low blood levels of DAO correlate to low gut levels of DAO—and gut levels are probably what matter most. Still, there is a limited amount of evidence that does indeed link low blood levels of DAO with symptoms of histamine intolerance, although there is no blood test that can definitively diagnose histamine intolerance. Interestingly, the placenta produces a substantial amount of DAO such that it is possible that pregnant people with histamine intolerance may experience a lessening of symptom severity!

There are also several medical conditions that can resemble histamine intolerance caused by DAO deficiency. Diseases and disorders that cause overproduction of histamine within your own body can overwhelm the body's capacity to degrade histamine, leading to histamine intolerance. Examples include severe seasonal and environmental allergies; **mast cell disorders**, or conditions that cause abnormally high numbers (or overactivity) of histamine-producing white blood cells called mast cells; excessive numbers of white blood cells called basophils, or **basophilia**; or histamine-releasing tumors called **carcinoid tumors**. People with these types of conditions will typically experience many more symptoms than just post-meal food intolerances, and will often have chronic, systemic symptoms that are quite debilitating and that are present whether or not they eat.

Some research suggests that the type of bacteria you harbor in your gut can contribute to an overload of histamine within the intestines and symptoms of histamine intolerance. Certain species are more likely to produce histamine than others, and people who harbor a relative abundance of histamine-producing overachievers may be more inclined to experience histamine intolerance than people who harbor fewer of them. In my clinical practice, I have similarly observed that a small subset of patients who were later found to have small intestinal bacterial overgrowth (or SIBO; see Chapter 6) initially presented to me with the telltale signs and symptoms of histamine intolerance. Upon successful treatment of their SIBO with antibiotics, the histamine intolerance resolved. In these cases, we've assumed that the excess bacteria they were overgrowing happened to be prolific histamine producers and were generating a higher-than-normal amount of histamine that was accumulating in the gut.

Another possible cause of histamine overproduction is caused by the use of opioid pain medications. When certain of these drugs are taken by mouth, they have been shown to trigger histamine release; indeed, itchiness is a very common side effect of pain medications like oxycodone, hydromorphone, or fentanyl. If you use any of these medications regularly, you may, have consistently elevated levels of histamine circulating in your blood, and this may render you more sensitive to the piling-on effect of meals that introduce additional histamine directly into your gut, which can make its way into the bloodstream. However, research into whether users of opioid pain medication actually experience histamine intolerance more than other groups of people is lacking. Similarly, many commonly used medications can suppress your normal levels of DAO, increasing the likelihood of histamine intolerance reactions. Clavulanic acid, a drug often added to antibiotics to improve their efficacy, is a potent DAO inhibitor. A blood pressure medication called verapamil also has a significant DAO-inhibiting effect. Amitriptyline, a tricyclic antidepressant and nerve pain medication that is widely prescribed for depression, migraines, IBS-D (and other functional GI disorders), and a variety of chronic pain disorders, also seems to have a moderate DAO-inhibiting effect.

How Diarrhea from Histamine Intolerance Presents

When a histamine reaction affects your digestive tract, you may experience any combination of the following symptoms within minutes to about an hour of eating the offending histamine-rich meal: abdominal pain, sudden-onset bloating, and/or diarrhea—which is often watery. The reaction doesn't last terribly long—usually no more than a few minutes (or a few trips to the bathroom) to a few hours—and in many cases, once it's over, you may go back to feeling perfectly fine as if nothing had happened (though this is not always the case). The bloating and/or diarrhea can sometimes be accompanied by any one of these other symptoms:

- Hives or itchy skin
- Swelling (angioedema), such as swelling lips, tongue, eyelids
- Feeling like your heart is racing (rapid heartbeat, or tachycardia)
- Tightening feeling in the throat or chest
- Acid reflux or heartburn
- Nausea
- Cloudy thinking or "brain fog"
- Fatigue immediately following a meal
- Headache (including migraines)
- Dizziness
- Runny nose or nasal congestion

In general, the reaction will happen soon after eating—particularly after eating high-histamine foods such as those listed in Table 8-1. If you are someone with a lot of seasonal allergies, these reactions may be more likely to happen at certain times of the year—like spring and/or fall allergy seasons—even if you are following your usual diet. Because of this, you may struggle to find any connection to specific food triggers. *After all*, you'll think to yourself, *I ate this same meal last month and it was totally fine!*

Relatedly, the total histamine load of a meal may also affect whether you react, meaning that a particular high-histamine food may be tolerated under some circumstances but cause a reaction in others. The minuscule amount of avocado contained in your California roll goes down without trouble, but you may then react to a larger portion of avocado when consumed as avo toast. Unless you know what you're looking for—or you enlist the help of a trained registered dietitian who does—you're not likely to figure out the food connection.

Diarrhea (and associated symptoms) from histamine intolerance typically does not respond to antidiarrheal medications or antispasmodic drugs. If you suspect you may be experiencing histamine intolerance, taking a dose of an antihistamine, such as Benadryl (diphenhydramine), can help provide proof of concept: if the diarrhea and any other digestive symptoms—like reflux, bloating, or stomach pain—go away quickly in response to an antihistamine medication, there's your answer.

It's important to note that histamine intolerance is NOT the same as a food allergy. Food allergies are adverse reactions to a food *protein* that is mounted by your immune system. Histamine intolerance reactions are not reactions to a food's protein but rather to the presence of histamine that's already present in the food. For example, a low-histamine dairy food like fresh milk should not trigger a histamine reaction in a histamine-intolerant person, but a high-histamine dairy food like aged Parmesan cheese is quite likely to. Similarly, super fresh (or flash-frozen) fish is well tolerated by most of my histamine-intolerant patients, but not-so-fresh fish? Not so much. Both contain the same proteins, but as you can see, the reaction is not triggered by the protein component of the food. Histamine intolerance reactions are *not* technically allergic reactions because the body's immune cells are not the source of the histamine, though many of the symptoms can certainly resemble one. (In fact, some of the research literature refers to them as pseudo-allergic reactions for precisely this reason.)

Diagnosing Histamine Intolerance

As of the time of this writing in late 2022, there are no objective, evidence-based lab tests available to diagnose a histamine intolerance. Rather, the diagnosis would be made clinically based on the presentation of symptoms in response to high-histamine foods, and their resolution with a low-histamine diet and/or antihistamine medications. A gastroenterologist or allergist/immunologist who stays current with the latest medical literature would be the right medical professional to seek out if you are experiencing symptoms that seem consistent with histamine intolerance. If you can, try to keep a food and symptom journal for two weeks (or longer) prior to your appointment, to help track patterns of what you eat and how it relates to any post-meal symptoms you experience. Record the time of all foods eaten and symptoms experienced, and also make note of whether you took any medications that day—particularly allergy medications. In evaluating you to determine possible causes of your symptoms, your doctor might conduct the following tests.

Food Allergy Testing

If you are having acute reactions after eating certain foods—particularly if those reactions involve more typical "allergic"-type symptoms like hives, itching, or acute diarrhea—your doctor will probably want to make sure you don't actually have a food allergy. Allergy testing may involve measuring blood levels of IgE antibodies to various foods to see if you are sensitized to any food proteins; this means that your body has flagged certain food proteins as foreigners and has started making some preparations to mount a future attack against them. Sensitization is a prerequisite to developing an allergy, though it does not automatically mean that you are allergic. In fact, only a small percentage of people who have been sensitized to a food protein actually go on to have allergic reactions to that food. Allergy testing may also include skin prick testing. In our practice, we've noticed that some people with suspected histamine intolerance may test negative for food allergies with skin prick testing . . . but will develop an enormous wheal in response to the histamine "control" that was scratched onto their skin. It is commonly the case for people with histamine intolerance to have no immune system sensitization to any food proteins, though many of our patients do have a number of seasonal and environmental allergies.

Blood and Urine Tests

At present, there is no blood test that's been validated to diagnose histamine intolerance—nor is there a breath test, urine test, gene test, or biopsy available, either. (I guess that's the trouble of being on the cutting edge of medical science!) However, there are blood tests that may help your doctor determine whether you may have other medical conditions that would predispose you to having an overload of histamine in your body that could make high-histamine foods harder to tolerate. Even if these come out negative, however, it does not rule out the possibility of your having an adverse reaction to a high-histamine food.

The doctors I work with most commonly check blood levels of histamine as well as levels of N-methylhistamine present in a 24-hour urine collection. These two tests may identify people whose bodies are overproducing histamine, presumably as the result of overactive mast cells. Doctors might also check your blood for an enzyme called tryptase, which is also secreted by mast cells, to see if it's abnormally high. If so, it may be an indication that those cells are overactive in a manner suggestive of a mast cell disorder; these are treated with a variety of medications—see below for more details. However, if you do not have a mast cell disorder underlying your histamine intolerance, your blood levels of histamine may be perfectly normal in between acute symptom attacks. For this reason, I have seen doctors create a standing order for histamine and tryptase blood work for my patients with suspected histamine intolerance issues, and instruct them to wait to have the blood drawn until their next symptom attack. The sooner you can get to a lab and have the blood taken in the aftermath of an episode, the more likely a doctor will be able to glimpse the fleeting evidence of elevated histamine levels as a contributing factor.

Some researchers have proposed that testing a person's blood levels of histamine before and then soon after giving them a medically supervised histamine challenge might be a better way to diagnose histamine intolerance. By comparing histamine levels at baseline with those after consuming a high-histamine food (or a dose of isolated pharmaceutical-grade histamine), a doctor may be able to detect evidence of an abnormal rise that would suggest some sort of buildup of histamine, as well as to observe whether (a) eating the food indeed provoked your usual symptoms, and (b) whether there was a correlation between onset of symptoms and blood levels of histamine. This approach has not yet been validated by the greater scientific community, nor is it common practice as of the time of this writing. However, there may be some pioneering doctors who are tinkering with this approach in their practices in an attempt to figure out what's at the root of their patients' symptoms.

A lab test that measures activity of the DAO enzyme in the blood is available online and through a growing number of labs that cater to functional/integrative practitioners and naturopaths, with many claiming it to be diagnostic for histamine intolerance. As of the time of this writing in late 2022, it has not been scientifically validated as a diagnostic marker, and it is not known whether having low levels of DAO in the blood necessarily means that someone will demonstrate symptoms of histamine intolerance. Based on available evidence, however, I imagine that it could be useful as one piece of data among many others in examining a person's overall situation in determining whether histamine intolerance seems to be a possibility.

Treating Histamine Intolerance

The central pillar of treatment for suspected histamine intolerance is the low-histamine diet, described below. Beware: The internet is brimming with versions of the low-histamine diet that contain wildly different information, most of which is unsubstantiated by reliable data. Medications and supplements may also help manage symptoms. Even though many of the medical remedies described below are available over the counter, I strongly encourage you to build your regimen under the supervision of a gastroenterologist or allergist/immunologist. These medications and supplements can all have side effects, and some should not be used along with others.

You should be monitored by a qualified, credentialed medical professional who is well trained in pharmacology—not a chiropractor, nutritionist, dietitian, or naturopath—if you're going to be using them regularly.

Medical Treatment for Histamine Intolerance

Antihistamines are medications that suppress histamine from affecting the tissues of the digestive system (and beyond); they fall into two categories: histamine-1 receptor (H_1) blockers and histamine-2 receptor (H_2) blockers. **H_1 blockers** prevent histamine from binding to receptors on mast cells, which release more histamine and other pro-inflammatory chemicals to the smooth muscle cells and other cells that line blood vessels—all of which are involved in allergic-type reactions. When histamine attaches to such receptors, it can produce symptoms like itching, headaches, heart racing, swelling, reduced blood pressure (that can cause dizziness), difficulty breathing or airway constriction, and pain. Examples of over-the-counter H_1 blocker medications include Claritin (loratadine), Zyrtec (cetirizine), Allegra (fexofenadine), and Xyzal (levocetirizine).

    H_2 blockers prevent histamine from binding to certain types of receptors on the specialized stomach cells that produce stomach acid as well as to receptors throughout the small intestine. Using these medications can reduce symptoms of heartburn and chest pain related to acid reflux that are triggered in some people with histamine intolerance, and in clinical practice, seem to improve tolerance to high-histamine foods when taken before meals. Examples of over-the-counter H_2 blocker medications include Pepcid and Zantac 360° (famotidine) and Tagamet (cimetidine). They are also available in prescription strength. Drugs like H_1 and H_2 blockers are typically used preventively to improve diet tolerance and reduce the likelihood of having a symptom attack.

    For acute-symptom attacks, however, first-generation antihistamine medications like Benadryl (diphenhydramine) are often used. Benadryl acts quickly to oppose the effects of histamine on the blood vessels, helping to quickly reduce the swelling-type reactions that can make breathing difficult or cause diarrhea in histamine intolerance. It can have more potential side effects than the other H_1 blockers described above, including drowsiness and constipation. For this reason, it's not a great choice for use as part of a daily regimen but rather best reserved for attacks of severe symptoms when your diet or other preventive regimen has failed. It's what I like to call a rescue remedy. You should not give Benadryl to children under the age of six unless directed to do so by their pediatrician.

DAO enzymes are also available to reduce post-meal symptoms of histamine intolerance. These are taken immediately before a meal. At present, only a few studies on DAO enzyme use in people with suspected histamine intolerance are available and have involved a cumulative total of fewer than two hundred people. In my clinical practice, I've had mixed results with it. I had one patient for whom it was an absolute miracle cure—enabling her to eat almost anything. Far more commonly, however, I see patients who feel it is a helpful tool that takes the edge off their post-meal symptoms and enables them to branch out from the low-histamine diet to a limited degree. There are also a fair number of my patients who try it out for a few weeks, don't notice much of a difference, and don't feel it's worth the effort or expense to keep taking. The best available data suggest that a dose of 4,000 HDU (that's histamine-digesting units) would be a reasonable place to start if you're interested in trying it out, though commercially available products typically contain between 10,000 and 20,000 HDU per pill.

You should note that currently marketed supplemental DAO is extracted from animals—pig kidneys, to be precise—and that the purity of such products sold as dietary supplements is not at all regulated by the US Food and Drug Administration (FDA). This manner of sourcing carries an inherent risk, though the DAO enzyme itself is considered quite safe assuming the animal from which it was derived was healthy. Plant-based sources of DAO have started to be commerialized but are less widely available. In the United States, the most widely available products are marketed by Omne Diem (Histamine Digest) and Seeking Health (Histamine Block). They cost about a dollar per capsule and are supposed to be taken about fifteen minutes before every meal.

If your doctor thinks your symptoms result from an overproduction of histamine by your own white blood cells rather than simply from lack of adequate DAO enzymes to break down dietary histamine (histamine intolerance), they may recommend medications or supplements called **mast cell stabilizers**. The most common such prescription medication is called Gastrocrom (cromolyn sodium), and it works by inhibiting your mast cells from secreting too much histamine. It is typically taken before eating and is available in a pill form, liquid drops, a nasal spray, or an inhaled nebulizer. Like all medications, it can have nontrivial side effects, so you should discuss these with your doctor if you are considering it.

A dietary supplement that is available over the counter, called quercetin, also seems to have mast cell–stabilizing effects—at least in laboratory tests—and is sometimes used to similar effect. Quercetin is an antioxidant that occurs naturally in certain fruits and vegetables—especially red wine, onions, and apple skins. There are some safety concerns with using high doses (more than 1 gram per day) of quercetin—specifically related to the risk of kidney damage. People with impaired kidney function and pregnant or nursing women should not take quercetin supplements. Most doctors I know who do recommend quercetin have their patients use it at doses of less than 1 gram daily for two weeks at a time, and then take a break from it for a little while before resuming use.

Dietary Treatment for Histamine Intolerance

The low-histamine diet is referenced constantly in research studies about histamine intolerance, but wildly different versions of this diet appear to be in circulation—few of which cite any original data sources to enable validation. It is extremely difficult to obtain reliable data on what foods are high in histamine, and the lists provided below reflect my best research into the deepest depths of the available data on the histamine content of food, which is scattered throughout decades-old books and obscure biochemistry journals. This task is complicated by the reality that histamine levels of a food will vary widely depending on its age, processing methods, and storage conditions. For this reason, I encourage you to use the lists below as a starting point for your low-histamine diet, and continue to keep track of your food and symptoms in a journal to help identify whether other foods may be giving you trouble beyond those listed here.

Table 8-1: High-Histamine Foods

Vegetables Naturally High in Preformed Histamine	Avocado
	Eggplant
	Red/ripe tomatoes (and tomato products like tomato juice, tomato paste, tomato sauce, etc.)
	Spinach
Aged, Cultured, Cured, and Fermented Foods	Asian condiments: black bean paste, fish sauce, gochujang, miso paste/soup, oyster sauce, soy sauce/tamari. . .
	Buttermilk, kefir, lassi drinks, sour cream, yogurt
	Cured/aged meats: dry sausages, pepperoni, prosciutto, salami
	Dry-aged steaks
	Fermented beverages: beer, hard apple cider, kombucha, kvass, wine (especially red wine)
	Fermented or pickled vegetables: kimchi, pickles, sauerkraut
	Hard/aged cheeses, especially Asiago, blue cheese, Parmesan, pecorino, Roquefort. . . others likely as well
	Vinegar and condiments/foods that contain it (ketchup, mustard, salad dressings)

(continues)

Table 8-1 *(continued)*

Not-So-Fresh Fish	"Fresh" fish and seafood that is not exceptionally fresh, including shrimp
	Processed fish: canned, cured, dried/preserved, and smoked, for example: anchovies, bacalao/salted cod, canned tuna, lox, pickled herring, sardines, smoked mackerel
	Spoiled fish
Yeast Extract	Savory flavored chips or vegan "cheezes" that contain yeast extract as a flavoring ingredient
	Yeast extract as a food additive or in products such as Maggi sauce, Marmite, Oxo, Vegemite
Soy Foods	Edamame
	Soy milk, soy yogurt, soy-based "cheeses" (e.g., Tofutti)
	"Soy nuts" (dry roasted soybeans)
	Soy protein isolate concentrate (added to bars, powders, protein drinks, veggie burgers)
	Soybean flour
	Tempeh
	Tofu
Other	Bloody Marys, tomato juice
	Cod liver oil supplements
	Worcestershire sauce

Note: See references at the end of the book for sources used to compile this list of histamine-containing foods.

Choose the Freshest-Possible Meats/Fishes and Avoid Leftovers

Because histamine develops in protein foods as they age, a particular meal may be tolerated well on the day you cook it but then trigger symptoms when you attempt to eat the leftovers a day or more later. To prevent development of histamine to the greatest degree possible,

I recommend buying the freshest chicken or meat you can and then freezing any portions you don't plan on cooking that same day. Similarly, store any leftover protein-containing foods (including dishes with beans) immediately in the freezer if you plan to consume them as leftovers. Thaw in the microwave immediately before you plan to consume them. Leftover vegetables and grains will likely be fine if stored in the fridge and consumed within a day or two, even without freezing.

Fish and seafood spoils much more quickly than meat and poultry, and has the potential to give you more trouble. Be aware that the "fresh" seafood sold on ice at your supermarket or fishmonger may have actually been caught a few days earlier and held under refrigeration or on ice, developing increased levels of histamine with each passing hour. For this reason, I recommend buying flash-frozen or individually quick frozen (IQF) fish fillets from your supermarket instead of the (seemingly) fresh alternative. You'll recognize IQF fish as those individually shrink-wrapped fillets. It is processed and frozen immediately after being caught, meaning that it has had much less opportunity to develop histamine on its way to your dinner plate. My patients typically tolerate homemade IQF fish well, whereas ordering fish from restaurants is very hit-or-miss.

Avoid Foods with Artificial Food Coloring and Certain Preservatives

Many people who react to high-histamine foods seem also to have difficulty tolerating certain artificial food additives, though it is not clear why. It is hypothesized that these food additives may cause white blood cells to release histamine, though at present this is just a guess; there is no clear explanation for how they might do so. Nonetheless, common triggers appear to be artificial food coloring, particularly tartrazine (otherwise known as yellow food dye, FD&C Yellow 5, or azo dye); benzoate preservatives, such as sodium or potassium benzoate; sulfite preservatives; and/or potassium sorbate. These food additives are commonly used in a wide swath of processed foods and drinks—from breakfast cereals, chips, and frozen potato products to sodas, fruit juices, and dried fruit—and many other categories of products as well. Organic foods should not contain any of these additives, with the exception of sulfites, which are allowed in organic wine. (Though wine should be avoided anyway on the low-histamine diet.) Natural preservatives less likely to trigger a reaction in sensitive people include vitamin E (tocopherol) and ascorbic acid (vitamin C). Natural food coloring from annatto, turmeric, beta carotene, beet powder, and purple carrot juice should also be well tolerated.

Limit Alcohol Intake

Alcohol inhibits the DAO enzyme required to degrade histamine within the body. Wine in particular typically contains preservatives called sulfites, which can trigger histamine reactions in some people as well, whereas beer and wine are also inherently high in histamine from their respective yeasty and bacterial fermentation processes. For these reasons, alcohol can be particularly problematic for people with histamine intolerance. However, some people do tolerate moderate amounts of clear spirits like vodka, gin, or tequila reasonably well, particularly when mixed with simple, low-histamine mixers like club soda or a cranberry juice cocktail.

Watch Out for Probiotic Supplements, and Consider Getting Tested for SIBO

It has been reported that certain strains of bacteria—including several in the *Lactobacillus* species—are particularly prolific producers of histamine. If you suspect you may be suffering from a histamine intolerance, it may be prudent to avoid using probiotics—particularly those containing *Lactobacillus* (sometimes listed on a label as an italicized capital "L." followed by a Latin strain name, such as *L. delbrueckii*). While some enterprising practitioners market probiotic supplements that purport to contain strains that actually degrade histamine in the gut and reduce symptoms of histamine intolerance, there's no convincing evidence (at least, not yet) to support these claims.

In my clinical practice, I've come across a few cases where patients appeared to develop a histamine intolerance characterized by bloating, cramping, and diarrhea following consumption of high-histamine foods. Further diagnostic testing revealed that these patients actually had small intestinal bacterial overgrowth, or SIBO (see Chapter 6). Once they were treated for their SIBO, the histamine intolerance resolved. If I had to guess, I'd say that these patients may have been overgrowing particular species of bacteria that produced high amounts of histamine, leading to excess amounts in the gut. Consuming high-histamine foods may have caused them to exceed their threshold for tolerance. I look forward to seeing whether research eventually emerges to account for these unusual cases! In the meantime, it's not a terrible idea to seek out noninvasive breath testing for SIBO if you've been afflicted with an apparent histamine intolerance somewhat out of the blue.

Choose Low-Histamine Foods as the Basis of Your Diet

While the table above emphasized foods to avoid, there are plenty of foods that should be well tolerated among people with histamine intolerance. The list below offers a starting point for your low-histamine diet, but tolerance is not guaranteed. Pay attention to whether certain foods on this list seem to aggravate your symptoms and individualize your diet accordingly.

If a food does not appear either on the high- or the low-histamine diet lists provided in this chapter, it either indicates a lack of available data about that food or it's a food for which available information is conflicting. Examples of such foods include strawberries, pineapple, citrus fruits (including lemon juice), cherries, plums, kiwi, mushrooms, chocolate, and pork. I recommended avoiding such foods for the first two weeks of your low-histamine diet. If your symptoms improve on the strictest version of this diet, you can begin introducing them and see how your body responds.

Table 8-2: Low-Histamine Foods

Fruits*	Apple Apricot Blueberries Coconut Fig Lychee fruit Mango Melon (all varieties) Peach Pear Starfruit *Avoid dried versions of these fruits if they are treated with sulfites as a preservative. Look for "sulfite-free" labels.
Vegetables	Asparagus Beets Broccoli Brussels sprouts Cabbage Carrots Cauliflower Corn Cucumber Garlic Green beans/string beans Kale Lettuces (all) Onions Potatoes Sweet potatoes/yams
Grains	All grains should be OK with the possible exception of bleached/bromated white (wheat) flour Choose whole wheat foods or organic white flour–based foods when possible if consuming wheat. Couscous and pasta made with durum and/or semolina flour should also be OK.

Table 8-2 *(continued)*

Proteins (All Fish, Meat, and Poultry Should Be Fresh or Immediately Frozen)	All beans, chickpeas, and lentils (except soybeans) All nuts (including nut butters like peanut butter) All seeds Eggs Flash-frozen or individually quick frozen (IQF) fish fillets Fresh beef (not dry aged) Poultry Pure hemp protein or rice protein powder without artificial coloring or sweeteners
Dairy Foods	Butter Cheeses that have not been bacterially fermented: cottage cheese, fresh mozzarella, mascarpone, natural cream cheese without added gums or stabilizers, paneer, ricotta cheese Cream, half-and-half Milk Natural gelato or vanilla ice cream without artificial ingredients or gums/stabilizers (e.g., Ciao Bella, Häagen-Dazs)
Beverages	Club soda Coffee Herbal teas (avoid "zests" and "zingers") Juice or nectars from low-histamine fruits Milk
Other/Misc:	All herbs and spices except possibly anise, chili powder, cinnamon, cloves, curry powder, nutmeg, pepper, salt Butter Chives, garlic, onion, scallions Oils Sugar (corn syrup, honey, maple syrup)

A Sample Day on the Low-Histamine Diet

While there are a variety of low-histamine fruits, veggies, grains, proteins, and seasonings to choose from, I'll be honest: it's still very difficult to eat out on a low-histamine diet. This is because you have no visibility into how fresh a restaurant's meat is; what individual seasonings are used in mixed dishes and sauces; and whether ingredients are sourced from brands that contain a variety of artificial preservatives. For these reasons, preparing most of your meals at home may be necessary to ensure relatively close adherence to the diet—particularly in the all-important first two weeks or so when you're trying to determine whether dietary histamine intake is actually triggering your diarrhea. In the chart below, I tried to include some foods that can be customized to be low-histamine when eating out (salads and smoothies) as well as some brands of convenience foods when available.

Table 8-3: A Sample Day on the Low-Histamine Diet

Meal	Sample Plant-Based Menu	Sample Omnivore Menu	Sample Paleo-Style Menu	Sample Gluten-Free Menu
Breakfast	Smoothie: Almond or coconut milk Banana Frozen mango Ground flaxseeds Hemp protein powder Honey or maple syrup to taste + Coffee with coconut milk	Hard-boiled egg Wasa wholegrain rye crispbreads topped with fig jam and peanut butter + Coffee with milk or half-and-half	Applegate Naturals Savory Turkey Breakfast Sausage Sliced melon + Coffee with coconut milk	Blueberries Maple buckwheat flakes cereal + milk (or coconut milk) + Coffee with milk or half-and-half
Lunch	Bay leaf Carrots Celery Garlic Lentils Onions Oregano Salt Water + Plain whole-grain crackers (like Triscuits) or rice	Baked or mashed potatoes with butter/salt (no cheese or sour cream added) Fresh rotisserie chicken Green beans	Baked salmon with garlic/olive oil/salt (Homemade from IQF fish; see discussion above) Riced cauliflower Sautéed garlic/kale	Salad topped with tahini dressing*: Arugula/Lettuce Beets Black beans Carrot Corn Cucumber Hard-boiled egg and/or fresh mozzarella cubes Sunflower seeds

(continues)

Table 8-3 *(continued)*

Meal	Sample Plant-Based Menu	Sample Omnivore Menu	Sample Paleo-Style Menu	Sample Gluten-Free Menu
Dinner	Quinoa bowl with: Arugula, Chickpeas, Corn, Cucumber, Sautéed zucchini, Tahini dressing*	Garlic/olive oil/pasta tossed with: Broccoli/broccoli rabe, Red pepper flakes, Ricotta cheese, White beans	Asparagus, Baked sweet potato, Steak (not dry aged)	Broccoli, Brown rice, Simple roasted chicken with olive oil/pepper/salt
Snack(s) and Treats	Apple/peanut butter, Ciao Bella Mango Sorbet, Hail Merry Coconut Vanilla Crème Miracle Tart, Popcorn	Carrots/hummus/tortilla chips, Ciao Bella Vanilla Gelato, KIND Healthy Grains bar in Oats & Honey flavor, Pear and almonds	Chia Pod (Banana, Blueberry, Mango) or coconut chia pudding (flavored with banana, honey, mango, and/or vanilla), Plantain chips/almond butter, Unsulfured dried mango, RXBAR Blueberry or Maple Sea Salt flavored	Dry roasted chickpeas (plain/salted), KIND Nuts & Spices bar in Madagascar Vanilla Almond or Maple Glazed Pecan flavors, Melon, Nature's Bakery Gluten Free Fig Bars

*To make tahini dressing, mix ¼ cup tahini paste with ½ tsp. ground cumin, ¼ tsp. kosher salt, 1 crushed garlic clove, and enough hot water to thin out the mixture to a dressing consistency.

Case Study: The Irritable Bowel Syndrome That Wasn't Irritable Bowel Syndrome

Yolanda was a thirty-year-old woman referred to me by her gastroenterologist for IBS, and her main complaint was the sudden appearance of severe attacks of diarrhea seven months earlier. While Yolanda had a lifelong history of "stomach issues," they had previously taken the form of constipation and had responded well to a simple laxative regimen. This whole diarrhea thing was completely new and foreign to her.

Yolanda described a situation in which she would experience a sudden, urgent need to defecate, and it resulted in four to five trips to the bathroom in a short period of time. The stool was loose and sometimes even watery. It could happen at any time of the day—and generally not in the mornings after waking up. Often, it would happen in the middle of a meal or very soon after. She recalled times of feeling the need to go on her way home from work so badly that she'd run into the front door and race to the toilet, still wearing her coat as she sat down to go. In between attacks, however, her bowel patterns were completely normal. Some days, she'd have normal, formed stools, or she might even skip a day of moving her bowels.

When I first saw Yolanda in January, her doctor had diagnosed the problem as IBS, having already ruled out celiac disease (Chapter 6) and inflammatory bowel disease (Chapter 7). She was prescribed some antispasmodic medication and sent my way. Based on the IBS diagnosis and Yolanda's typical dietary habits—she had a large kale salad for lunch almost daily—I proceeded to recommend soluble fiber therapy (Chapters 4, 12), advising her to avoid salads and other forms of "roughage," and to start taking a soluble fiber supplement like Citrucel.

I didn't hear from Yolanda again until May. Apparently, the soluble fiber therapy approach didn't really make a difference during the first two weeks she tried it. But no matter; soon after, her diarrhea disappeared as mysteriously as it had suddenly appeared, despite no change in her diet and resuming daily lunch salads. This honeymoon period lasted for a few months until the diarrhea came back once again in late April—worse than before.

At this point, Yolanda's doctor and I realized that we weren't dealing with garden-variety IBS anymore. We tried a low-FODMAP diet commonly prescribed for people with IBS (Chapter 4) and had her breath tested to rule out small intestinal bacterial overgrowth (SIBO, Chapter 6). The test was negative and the diet did nothing to alleviate her symptoms. In fact, Yolanda remarked that a few very high-FODMAP foods actually seemed to be among her safest ones: she could eat unlimited quantities of mango, watermelon, and brussels sprouts without provoking an attack. Running out of ideas, her doctor wondered whether Yolanda was experiencing bile acid diarrhea (Chapter 6) that was hitting her twelve or more hours after eating the offending food, making it difficult to connect the symptom with the trigger. But a trial of the medication used to treat bile acid diarrhea also had no effect on her symptoms.

The breakthrough came when Yolanda mentioned in passing that her seasonal allergies had been flaring terribly these past few weeks, and she had started to take a heavy-duty regimen of histamine-blocking medications to deal with them. That's when a light bulb finally went off. "You have seasonal allergies?" I asked. "Terrible ones," she replied. Suddenly, all the pieces came together. Yolanda's best-tolerated foods were all low-histamine ones, and she was currently flaring at the peak of spring allergy season. Previous trigger meals she had reported to me had all involved a high-histamine food: a roasted *tomato* caprese salad doused in *vinegar*, a Greek omelet with *spinach*, *tomato*, and *feta*; it was starting to seem quite likely that Yolanda was histamine intolerant.

I decided to try Yolanda on a low-histamine diet. She was completely better within days. I advised her to stay on this diet during the peak allergy seasons of spring and fall, and that she could try testing tolerance for higher-histamine favorites in the off-seasons of midwinter and the peak of summer, probably with the support of her usual histamine-blocking medication regimen. Then I referred her to a terrific allergist/immunologist, under whose care she continues to be. It's been years since I worked with Yolanda, and as far as I know, she's been regular ever since.

Yolanda's case illustrates some of the classic clues of histamine intolerance: a history of seasonal allergies; gastrointestinal symptoms that come and go at different times of the year, punctuated by completely normal intermissions; and complete lack of response to typical diet and medicine interventions for diarrhea. This is a diagnosis that is often arrived at after failure of multiple other treatment trials, and that is often mistakenly diagnosed as IBS. As for what I learned as a dietitian from Yolanda's case: always ask your patients about whether they have seasonal allergies!

PART III

Slow and Unsteady

Chronic Constipation

9

No Flow, No Go

Constipation from Fiber Imbalance

IF YOU'VE BEEN STRUGGLING WITH constipation for a long time, I imagine that at some point you've encountered the pretty standard advice to "eat more fiber," and you've possibly even tried to do so already. Still, no book about managing constipation could claim to be comprehensive without at least including some details about one of the most common causes of constipation, which is also the most straightforward one to treat: not eating enough dietary fiber to produce regular, complete bowel movements even though your colon's transit time may be completely normal. But not consuming enough fiber is only one type of fiber imbalance that can contribute to constipation; in some cases, eating too much of one type of fiber (insoluble) and not enough of another (soluble) can also be constipating in predisposed individuals. So, let's start at the beginning: What is fiber and how does it help us poop?

Fiber is a specific type of carbohydrate that is found exclusively in plant-based foods. By definition, there is no fiber in meat, chicken, fish, eggs, or dairy, and there is no fiber in foods that are 100% fat, such as oils, even if these oils come from plants. What makes fiber different from other types of carbohydrates, such as sugar or starch, is that human beings lack digestive enzymes that are capable of breaking apart the chemical bonds that hold fiber together. In other words, fiber is indigestible to humans.

The fact of fiber's indigestibility has two important results. First, unlike other carbohydrates, it has a negligible number of calories. If we can't break it down during digestion, then we can't extract the same amount of energy (calories) from fiber as we can from digestible carbohydrates like sugar or starch, which supply us with about four calories per gram. Because the fiber we eat is indigestible, it remains intact in our guts and travels all the way to the colon, which happens also to house trillions of bacteria that are collectively referred to as the gut microbiota. And this is where fiber's utility to us humans becomes apparent.

The fate of fiber in our colon will depend on what type of fiber it is. **Insoluble fiber** is the type of fiber we often think of as "roughage." It's a type of fiber that doesn't dissolve in water but rather stays pretty intact throughout its entire journey through the GI tract. It's the predominant type of fiber in leafy vegetables; fruit, vegetable, and bean skins; the tough outer coating of seeds; and nuts. Because it remains largely intact throughout its digestive journey, insoluble fiber is often the fiber that's visibly recognizable in your stool—the outer layer of corn kernels, the flaxseeds, the tomato skins, and the crumpled-up spinach leaves. Although it doesn't do a great job of feeding the gut bacteria, its bulkiness is the key to a different digestive benefit. Bulky insoluble fiber tends to push up against the intestinal walls, stimulating them to contract and keep things moving forward.

In contrast, the **soluble fiber** found in the flesh of fruits and squashes, root vegetables, grains, and the inside of beans *is* able to dissolve in water, and when it does, it forms a viscous gel that acts in a spongelike way. This type of fiber can hold on to moisture and make sure that stools don't get hard and dried out on their way through the colon; picture the absorption that happens when you leave soluble fiber–rich oats soaking in water for five minutes and you'll have a pretty good idea of how this fiber behaves in the gut. I think of soluble fiber as the glue that holds a poo together. In fact, this gooey, gluey attribute is a key way that eating soluble fiber–rich foods helps lower blood cholesterol levels and reduces the risk of cardiovascular disease: Dietary cholesterol we eat literally gets trapped in the goo and can't get absorbed into our bodies. This forces the liver to pull cholesterol out of the bloodstream in order to obtain an adequate supply for use in the body.

Some types of soluble fiber are also very **fermentable**. Fermentable means that gut bacteria are able to break apart its chemical bonds and digest it themselves, fueling their own growth (and often making some gas in the process). The prebiotic fibers and high-FODMAP foods discussed in Chapter 4 on IBS-D are all examples of fermentable fibers. A very small amount of energy (calories) is liberated in this fermentation process, which is why it's more accurate to say that fiber has a minimal number of calories per gram but technically not zero calories per gram. Our best estimates are that accessible calories from fermentable types of fiber range from one to two calories per gram, which is between 25% and 50% of a digestible carbohydrate like sugar or starch. This fact can help account for the observation that people whose diets are higher in fiber tend to have an easier time maintaining lower body weights compared with people whose diets are lower in fiber. Simply put: it's easier to keep daily calorie intake from going overboard when you are filling up on more foods that have one to two calories per gram compared with "regular" carbohydrates (4 calories/gram), protein (4 calories/gram), or fat (9 calories/gram).

As the descriptions above suggest, a healthy balance of both insoluble and soluble fiber helps keep us regular in the bathroom; see Table 12-2 in Chapter 12 for a list of foods that contain predominantly soluble fiber, and for a list of predominantly insoluble fiber–rich foods, see "Foods to Avoid or Modify on a Gentle Fiber Diet" in Chapter 12 on page 248.

Consuming soluble fiber makes sure our stools stay soft, formed, and cohesive, whereas consuming insoluble fiber helps contribute to bulkier stools that move along at a nice, healthy pace and don't require much muscle straining for us to pass. When people adopt very restrictive lower-carb diets—such as Whole30, keto, or Atkins—the balance of fiber usually skews heavily toward insoluble fiber from low-carb staples like salad, nuts, and berries, and intake of soluble fiber becomes relatively low. It's not at all unusual for this to result in constipation for some people! Lacking the water-retaining capacity of soluble fiber, stools can become hard and dried out.

Diagnosing Constipation Due to Fiber Imbalance

Many of my patients have an inkling that they're not getting enough fiber consistently when they report to me that eating an extra serving of fruit each day or having a salad a few times per week helps them go to the bathroom more regularly and/or more completely. Still, sometimes we get so busy—or our dietary habits start to gradually and subtly shift in ways we don't immediately notice—and we suddenly find ourselves pooping less without realizing why. Keeping an electronic food journal for a week, particularly one that automatically calculates fiber grams as you enter your foods—can be an easy way to audit whether fiber intake is likely the problem. If your average daily intake is below 20 grams, there's a reasonable chance that increasing fiber intake would be a helpful first place to start.

But what if you're not just regularly meeting these recommended intake levels, but are actually exceeding them, and your stools are still infrequent, hard, and/or incomplete? One thing to consider is the balance of different types of fiber in your diet. If you get most of your fiber from insoluble sources like salad, cooked leafy vegetables like spinach or kale, nuts, seeds, and berries—and you eat minimal foods like non-berry fruit, root veggies, whole grains, beans, or squashes—then it's possible that your relatively high-fiber diet isn't striking the fiber balance your gut needs to produce softer, more complete stools at frequent intervals. I see this happen a lot in my patients who choose to restrict calories and carbs on various weight-loss or so-called "clean-eating" diets. If your colon's transit time happens to be a little bit on the slower side, then a diet that's high in bulky insoluble fiber that can't hold on to much moisture and is devoid of spongy soluble fiber can sometimes result in stools that get hard and dried out as they take their sweet old time moving through your colon.

To be clear, this doesn't happen to everyone who adopts a low-carb diet. Plenty of people who adopt one of the veggie-rich low-carb diets described above actually report having an improvement in their bowel movements and overall regularity compared with their constipation-prone baseline. Some may even experience diarrhea! The point is that a drastic diet change can affect our unique bodies in different and often surprising ways, and patients who do find themselves feeling bloated and constipated despite *increasing* their daily fiber intake on a healthy new diet regimen are often quite shocked to learn that their seeming good deed was being punished in such a way. Sometimes the balance of the type of fiber you eat is as important as the total number of grams of fiber you eat. A simple bowl of soluble fiber–rich oatmeal and some mango, pear, or melon can go a very long way!

While my clinical nutrition practice is for adults and I don't consult with children, I do think it's worth mentioning that inadequate fiber intake is common among children, and studies confirm that children with low-fiber intakes are more likely to be constipated than children with higher-fiber intakes. Signs and symptoms of constipation from inadequate fiber in children can be a little different from that in adults. Chronic bellyaches are a really common one. In more severe cases of constipation, kids may have to pee more often than usual or even be prone to bed-wetting or daytime urinary incontinence (peeing accidents); this is because a colon full of stool can put pressure on the bladder and make it hard for kids to hold in their urine. A condition called **encopresis** may also affect chronically constipated children. Encopresis is a fancy way of saying pooping in the underpants; it's when smears or small blobs of soft stool leak out and stain the underwear, and it's akin to the phenomenon of overflow diarrhea in adults that I described in Chapter 2. Another sign of encopresis is that your child may be prone to passing large-diameter stools that actually clog the toilet, especially after several days of not going at all.

Treating Constipation
Due to Fiber Imbalance

The treatment for constipation due to fiber imbalance is far more dietary than it is medical, and is described in the following section. Nonetheless, there are some inexpensive, safe, over-the-counter remedies that you can employ in the event that you struggle to keep up with your fiber intake consistently enough to stay regular in the bathroom.

Fiber supplements are safe and effective for both adults and children, and can be very helpful in regulating bowel movements by ensuring a consistent, concentrated dose of moisture-holding, stool-bulking fiber. While fiber supplements don't have the same overall health benefits as dietary fiber from whole foods and should not be a substitute for working toward adequate dietary intake, they can certainly help regulate the form, consistency, and frequency of your bowel movements. If you are on a low-carb diet lacking in soluble fiber–rich foods and are unwilling to expand your diet to include more carbs, then a fiber supplement may be necessary to offset the effect of fiber imbalance in your diet.

A variety of fiber supplement types have been demonstrated to be helpful in relieving constipation, and they are marketed in powder, pill, and gummy forms. For constipation, I tend to recommend more bulking varieties of fiber that have high water-holding capacity, such as psyllium (marketed as Metamucil and Konsyl) or calcium polycarbophil (marketed as FiberCon); for people who prefer pills, an effective dose of FiberCon is typically just two pills, whereas it can take up to five pills of psyllium to achieve the same benefits. Fiber supplements absolutely must be taken along with a full glass of water to be effective. As my gastroenterologist colleague Dr. Eric Goldstein famously tells his patients, "If you supplement fiber without enough water, you'll make bricks, not poops."

Over-the-counter medications that help attract water into the bowel can also be helpful remedies for too-hard stools as you work to get your fiber intake perfected. These are called **osmotic laxatives** and include MiraLAX (polyethylene glycol), Phillips' Milk of Magnesia (a form of magnesium called magnesium hydroxide), or just regular old magnesium from the vitamin aisle taken in doses between 400 and 1,000 mg. People with kidney disease should contact their doctor before taking magnesium. If you take a too-high dose of an osmotic laxative, your stools will be loose or you may even get diarrhea, which is your cue to reduce the dose and try again. I typically recommend dosing these laxatives at night if you wish to move your bowels in the morning.

Dietary Management of Constipation Due to Fiber Imbalance

While there is no single magic amount of fiber that will guarantee you regularity as an individual, we do have some general guidelines about what adequate fiber intake levels are for the population on an average level. You may require a bit more or even a bit less than these numbers to stay regular in the bathroom and live your healthiest, most comfortable life. Both the National Academy of Medicine and the Dietary Guidelines for Americans, 2020–2025, advise that an adequate intake of fiber would be 14 grams for every 1,000 calories in our diets. This is where the general advice that **women should consume at least 25 g of fiber per day and men should consume 38 g of fiber per day** comes from; these numbers assume that the average woman consumes about 1,800 calories per day, and the average man is consuming about 2,700 calories per day. These numbers are guidelines, not prescriptions. An adequate amount of fiber for you personally may be more or less than this, and a tolerable amount of fiber for you may be more or less than this.

Nonetheless, it's safe to say that most Americans fall far short of these guidelines. An analysis of population-level data between the years 1999 and 2010 found that the average fiber intake among US adults is about 16 to 17 g per day; women consumed about 14 g per day and men about 18 g per day. While this particular data set did not suggest any difference in average fiber intake between younger adults and older adults on average, I will say anecdotally that I do find some of my elderly patients can be especially prone to constipation caused by inadequate fiber intake. When older people live alone, lose a spouse, or simply feel too tired or unmotivated to bother with grocery shopping and cooking, they often default to simple, low-effort meals that lack fiber-rich fruits, vegetables, and legumes. Having dental issues that render chewing difficult can also predispose a diet toward softer, simpler foods like eggs, toast, turkey sandwiches, cereal, canned soups, chicken and rice, burgers, pasta . . . none of which have much fiber to speak of.

There's a bit less consensus around fiber guidelines for children; I typically use the guidelines put forth by the American Academy of Pediatrics (AAP) of "age plus 5 to 10 grams" as a good general target, though the National Academy of Medicine has set guidelines far higher than this. As a parent to school-age children myself, I recognize how challenging it can be to ensure that kids meet their fiber needs consistently. Having a dietitian mom doesn't bestow an innate love of kale in a child, and despite having been routinely presented with a variety of nuts, seeds, beans, veggies, fruits, and whole-grain foods since being weaned to solid foods, my own children are only self-motivated to consume a more limited number of these foods than I would hope for. As kids get older, parents also lose the ability to control what foods they have access to for the many hours they're away from us, and I know for a fact that many of the fiber-rich snacks I pack in lunchboxes get traded away for the low-fiber, pirate-themed puffed corn snacks I've refused to buy. (At least someone's kid is eating the fiber, I suppose!)

I think it's important to also aim for a balance in the types of fiber you consume to optimize bowel function. Going for the number of grams without thought to the quality and type of fiber you consume may not produce the results you're seeking. You may be able to reach 25 g of fiber per day without eating a single fruit, vegetable, whole grain, nut, or bean if you were to eat one low-carb

Quest bar (17 g fiber) and a pint of Halo Top ice cream (12 g fiber), but I'm betting you may wind up bloated, gassy as all get-out, and not necessarily even pooping any better. If you're serious about your digestive health beyond just getting a decent poop out each day, there are no shortcuts or ways around the need to eat a diversity of actual, real plant foods.

Table 9-1: Sample Balanced Fiber Diets for All Types of Eaters

	Sample Menu for People Who Don't Cook at All	Sample Fiber-Rich Kid-Friendly Menu	Sample Menu for Carb-Conscious Eaters
Breakfast	Packet of Nature's Path Flax Plus instant oatmeal, made in microwave, topped with: Blueberries (fresh or frozen) Sliced almonds Sweetened (or not) to taste	Almond flour pancakes (look online for Elana's Pantry Silver Dollar Pancakes recipe) Strawberries Syrup of choice	1 slice Ezekiel bread Eggs Mashed avocado
Lunch	Chipotle Burrito Bowl with: Black or pinto beans Brown rice (optional) Fajita vegetables Hot sauce or other salsas of choice Lettuce Meat/protein of choice Roasted chili corn salsa	Lunchbox: 88 Acres Seed & Oat bar (nut-free) or KIND bar mini (contains nuts) Grapes Popcorn Sandwich of choice on wholegrain white bread (e.g., Pepperidge Farm Farmhouse)	Baked salmon Riced cauliflower Sautéed string beans with slivered almonds

(continues)

Table 9-1 *(continued)*

	Sample Menu for People Who Don't Cook at All	Sample Fiber-Rich Kid-Friendly Menu	Sample Menu for Carb-Conscious Eaters
Dinner	Order-in Chinese meal as follows: Stir-fried medley of veggies (e.g., bok choy, broccoli, carrots, onion, snow peas, string beans) . . . with chicken or shrimp or tofu Order brown or garlic sauce on the side Substitute brown rice instead of white	Buttered broccoli with Parmesan cheese Chicken or meat of choice Corn on the cob + Dessert: frozen smoothie popsicles	Chicken or turkey meatballs No-sugar-added tomato sauce Spiralized zucchini "noodles"
Snack(s) and Treats	Apple, clementines Hummus with baby carrots Microwave popcorn Smoothie from a local juice bar—choose one that is mostly fruit and/or greens	Banana/berry fruit smoothie; pour 2 TBSP chia seeds into the blender Beanitos brand tortilla chips + guacamole Happy Herbert's Spelt Snack Sticks Homemade carrot and zucchini mini muffins (use Giada De Laurentiis's recipe available online)	Chia pudding made with unsweetened plant-based milk of choice with added raspberries Edamame Hummus with baby carrots KIND Nuts & Spices bar

Case Study:
Raine's Lower-Carb Diet Debacle

Raine was referred to me by her gastroenterologist with a variety of issues she needed to address. She had a long-standing history of both constipation as well as acid reflux, and had been on proton pump inhibitor (PPI) medications for years to control the latter. The combination of her backed-up bowels and long-standing acid-suppressing medication use seemed to have created perfect conditions for Raine to overgrow bacteria in her small intestine, as she had been diagnosed with—and treated for—SIBO (Chapter 6) just prior to meeting with me. Raine also had type 2 diabetes and recently her blood sugars had been trending higher than usual. She was looking for dietary solutions that would help manage both her constipation and blood sugars to prevent her SIBO from returning and get her diabetes back under control. Her doctor had her taking magnesium supplements to help her move her bowels more regularly until she had a chance to meet with me to discuss diet.

A quick spin through Raine's usual diet showed that she was trying to be carb conscious for her diabetes and limit portions of grains and starches. In so doing, though, she was defaulting to low-fiber, protein-rich options like eggs and turkey bacon for breakfast, or Greek yogurt as a snack. To address her constipation, though, Raine was relying heavily on consuming dried fruits like prunes, raisins, and apple chips—which were probably too much concentrated sugar at once given her blood sugar issues. There was a good portion of salad or cooked spinach with dinner every night and a handful of nuts in the afternoon, but clearly it wasn't enough to keep Raine regular. These lower-carb fiber sources were predominantly insoluble fiber, and she probably needed a better balance of foods with soluble fiber and insoluble fiber to regulate her bowel patterns.

Tweaking the amount, type, and food sources of fiber in Raine's diet was therefore the focus of my recommendations. Her tendency toward lower-carb eating was resulting in not enough fiber overall, and her avoidance of even high-fiber grains or legumes that would

have a modest impact on her blood sugar in favor of relatively lib-
eral amounts of dried fruit wasn't the best trade-off in terms of blood
sugar control. I had Raine ease off the dried fruit and introduce some
modest portions of lower-glycemic carbs like steel-cut oats, fresh
berries, bean salads, lentil soups, and sweet potato to her breakfasts
and lunches, and I also encouraged adding some other options like
ground flaxseeds and soluble fiber–rich avocado on most days as well.

Within two weeks on a higher-fiber diet as described above,
Raine was moving her bowels fully and easily at least once per day—
sometimes even twice—and no longer needed magnesium supplements as a laxative. Around the same time, some motility test results
came back (see Chapter 10 for descriptions), which showed that
the transit time through every segment of Raine's digestive system
was completely normal. In other words, Raine had been experiencing "normal transit" constipation, whereby her bowel motility was
working perfectly fine; she just wasn't consuming enough fiber to
stay regular! Not only did Raine's higher and more balanced fiber
diet help get her regular without the need for laxatives, but it also
resulted in a few pounds of weight loss. Three months later, her
blood sugar levels were much improved as well.

*

What if you already eat loads of fiber and *still* NOTHING comes
out? In fact, what if a high-fiber diet makes you feel *more* bloated
and constipated, not less? Skip ahead to Chapter 11, "Constipation
by Outlet Dysfunction."

Slow Motility

IBS-C and Slow Transit Constipation

IT CAN SOMETIMES SEEM LIKE splitting hairs when we talk about the many different causes of constipation, but there are important differences why any two given people may not be able to move their bowels regularly, completely, and easily. Understanding the underlying causes is essential for targeted treatment. For example, constipation caused by lack of fiber or imbalanced fiber may occur in people whose colons work perfectly well and are not slow or sluggish in the least. And as the following chapter on outlet dysfunction will explain, some people with perfectly normal colonic transit time can still find themselves terribly constipated as a result of problems with the nerves and muscles responsible for coordinating around the actual act of defecation. It's sort of like arriving on time to the airport gate but finding the door jammed, and you completely miss your flight anyway. This chapter will address the diagnosis and management of forms of constipation caused by irregular motility (movement) or slow movement patterns within the intestines.

Irritable Bowel Syndrome (IBS-C) and Slow Transit Constipation

The main difference between regular **slow transit constipation** and **constipation-predominant irritable bowel syndrome (IBS-C)** has to do with how much pain you experience. While people with many types of constipation may have similar-looking stool (e.g., hard balls or hard lumpy sausages that align to Bristol type 1 to type 3 references on the Bristol Stool Chart shared in Chapter 2) and may even move their bowels with similar degrees of frequency (or infrequency), people with IBS are generally experiencing a greater degree of pain overall.

As I explained in Chapter 4, a central characteristic of all subtypes of IBS is an over-sensation of pain in response to stimuli within the gut. This is called **visceral hypersensitivity**. (If you're interested in what causes this hypersensitivity, flip back to page 47 for an explanation on the gut-brain axis and the various gut hormones and neurotransmitters that play a role in it.) For this reason, people with IBS-C may be treated with additional medications that seek to address hypersensitive nerves and/or pain perception communication channels between the gut and the brain. These are detailed later in the chapter. This facet of IBS-C may also have implications for dietary remedies; certain foods that generate more stimulating sensations in the gut—from coarse, bulky fiber (think kale salad) to typically gassy forms of fiber (think beans and brussels sprouts) may be better tolerated in people with standard slow transit constipation than in people with IBS-C.

How Do Symptoms of IBS-C and Slow Transit Constipation Present?

My patients with both forms of constipation often tell me that when they're "doing everything right"—keeping up with a high-fiber diet, exercising regularly, drinking coffee each morning, drinking plenty of water throughout the day, and getting enough sleep—then it helps improve their constipation to a modest degree, but things are still never objectively great. They often do respond well to over-the-counter laxatives like MiraLAX, magnesium, senna, or Dulcolax (bisacodyl) but find it frustrating that they can't have regular or complete-enough stools without having to take something. Sometimes patients complain that they don't have urges to go at all without using some sort of laxative, and many resist using these regularly for fear of "becoming dependent." Bowel movements can feel disappointingly incomplete. There is often a fair amount of farting, and this is typically worse at night. Often, they also complain of chronic bloating or a visibly distended lower abdomen that is flattest in the morning (but rarely actually flat), temporarily flatter after pooping, but then it can build back up quite a bit by the end of the day.

People with IBS-C may have the additional complaint of experiencing pain after meals, especially larger meals or higher-fiber meals. Pain may be dull or crampy, and it's only alleviated if they can have a bowel movement—which oftentimes they cannot. With IBS-C, patients also sometimes describe that the severity of their constipation can vary based on their level or amount of stress, anxiety, and sleep. Bowel function may be worse when stressed or anxious and mildly better when relaxed, but things are still not objectively good even when stress levels are low.

Diagnosing IBS-C and Slow Transit Constipation

When you come in for your first visit complaining of constipation, most doctors aren't usually going to offer an extensive series of invasive tests before seeing how you respond to some basic, safe interventions. Chances are, they'll suggest some combination of a high-fiber diet, MiraLAX, and/or (much to my dismay) a random probiotic of some sort. Some docs will also tell you to drink lots of water, as if you haven't already tried that, which, frankly, is probably not the expert advice you were hoping to get when you booked this doctor's appointment six weeks ago and paid a forty-dollar co-payment for the visit.

A thorough doctor will also take the time to review your medical history, family history, and medication list to see if there are any likely culprits that could be underlying your constipation—especially if the problem is a newer one for you. To make sure you get a thorough evaluation like this, I'd advise you to provide a written list of all medications and dietary supplements you take, as well as a summary list of all medical conditions you have. If there is a family history of colon cancer or thyroid disease, it would be prudent to mention that as well.

But assuming your medication list and health history don't contain any smoking guns, and conservative measures such as fiber and MiraLAX don't produce sufficient relief, your doctor may order some additional diagnostic tests to dig deeper into what, precisely, they are dealing with and to help inform an appropriate treatment.

Blood Work

IBS is typically a clinical diagnosis that's made on the basis of reported symptom patterns once organic diseases like celiac disease or inflammatory bowel disease have been ruled out. Therefore, your doctor may start with some basic blood work to rule these out. They may also check your thyroid-stimulating hormone (TSH) levels to make sure you don't have hypothyroidism, which can cause constipation, or hypercalcemia (high blood calcium), which can come from a variety of illnesses and also cause constipation.

Colonoscopy

There's a reasonable chance that your doctor may order a colonoscopy at some point, especially if the constipation is a new symptom and/or you are over forty years old. This is because new-onset constipation can be a symptom of colon cancer, and your doctor will want to be sure to rule it out. However, the vast majority of constipation cases are not caused by cancer, and therefore colonoscopy alone rarely provides a diagnosis about the cause of your issue. Even so, the pre-procedure colon cleanout might bring some welcome relief to your chronically backed-up bowel, and the peace of mind should bring psychological, if not physiological, relief.

Motility Studies

Assuming your blood work is unremarkable and your response to over-the-counter laxative remedies is unsatisfactory, your doctor might decide to pursue motility testing. (Though they may skip right ahead to a trial of a prescription medication, described later in this chapter.) A variety of multiday tests are available to help your doctor measure how long it takes food and waste to move through your digestive tract and see (1) whether you have slow transit, and (2) if so, how slow it is. These tests work by sending identifiable markers through your GI tract and measuring how your transit time compares to expected reference ranges in order to diagnose slow transit constipation.

One such study is called a **Sitz marker test**. This entails you swallowing a capsule that contains tiny markers that can be tracked via X-ray as they make their way through your colon. You will return to the radiologist's office for an X-ray a few days after swallowing the pill to see if any of the little markers remain—and possibly a second time. It's important to recognize, however, that a Sitz marker test can be abnormal in about 50% of people who have **outlet dysfunction** constipation (Chapter 11), though people constipated due to **pelvic floor dysfunction** will often demonstrate different patterns on a Sitz marker test from people constipated due to slow transit. Still, if you have any suspicious symptoms of pelvic floor or anorectal muscle dysfunction, it may be worth asking your doctor whether it makes sense to start with a different diagnostic test (called anorectal manometry) that examines pelvic floor muscle function; the test is described in Chapter 11. These symptoms include straining to poop even when your stools are perfectly soft; extremely infrequent bowel movements; occasional fecal incontinence (stool leaks or slips out by accident); anal pain; lack of any response to even high-dose laxatives; painful sexual intercourse; and/or urinary problems. See Chapter 11 for more information about this type of constipation.

Another type of motility study called **transenteric scintigraphy** provides more extensive data about transit times throughout the entire digestive tract—stomach, small intestine, and colon. Sometimes your doctor will order such a test if they suspect you may have more global motility problems that affect you in ways beyond just constipation. For example, if you have upper digestive symptoms, this test can rule out slow stomach emptying; if you have recurrent bouts of small intestinal bacterial overgrowth (SIBO; Chapter 6), this test can see if your small intestine's transit time is delayed; and it will also see how long things take to move through your colon as well. This is a multiday test that has you in a radiologist's office for six hours on the first day, consuming a test meal of radiolabeled food (yum!). You will return each day for the next three days for a quick photo using a specialized camera.

More specialist gastroenterology practices may offer an alternative method of whole-gut motility testing called the **SmartPill**, which is a single-use pill that contains sensors that wirelessly transmit data to a device you'll wear around your neck or waist (or keep very close by) for the duration of the test. It records data on how long the capsule spends in each section of the digestive tract, and other potentially useful information as well, including pH levels, temperature, and muscle pressure. It's a less time-consuming process for you, as you'll just need to show up to the doctor's office, eat a special bar, and swallow the pill before going on your merry way. Once you poop out the capsule—usually within three to five days— the test is over and you can return the recorder device to your doctor so they can download the data. However, some doctors may still prefer transenteric scintigraphy, as it provides more geographic data within the small bowel and colon, and also because the SmartPill study does not pick up signs of pelvic floor dysfunction well.

Pelvic Floor Function Tests

If you continue to struggle with constipation despite various medications, and blood or motility tests don't turn up helpful answers, your doctor may order one or more tests that evaluate the function of various muscles involved in defecation. Examples are **anorectal manometry** and **MR defecography**. These are explained in detail on pages 226–227 in Chapter 11.

Treating IBS-C and Slow Transit Constipation

Medical Approaches for Managing IBS-C and Slow Transit Constipation

While there is no cure for IBS, there are numerous over-the-counter and prescription medication options that are effective at helping people increase the frequency of their bowel movements, improve stool consistency and reduce pain associated with defecation or the urge to defecate. It can take a bit of experimentation to land on a **bowel regimen** that produces the right balance of results for you, so once you've unlocked the magic combination, it's important to stay consistent! A bowel regimen is just a technical term we use to describe the toileting routines and medications or supplements a person employs to help maintain regularity.

Many of my patients resist the idea that they need to rely on a laxative to help them stay regular, and will use it for a while until their bowel patterns normalize. Then, the magical thinking takes over and they convince themselves that their bowels have somehow learned how to function normally on their own during this period of laxative use and stop taking their medications or supplements consistently. Sure enough, the bowels revert back to their baseline levels of function once the bowel regimen is withdrawn. To be clear, your *dependence* on these medications is different from building a *tolerance* to these medications. This is to say that using these medications won't make your baseline motility any worse than it already is, even if you use them regularly for a long time. And once you identify an effective dose of these meds, you won't need to keep ratcheting it up, because your body shouldn't "get used" to them and become impervious to their effects. If you're not able to move your bowels well without some extra support, I would argue that you're already *dependent* on this support whether or not you choose to use it. So why not use the tools available to you so you can feel better?

Over-the-Counter Laxatives

There are two main modes of action for over-the-counter laxatives: **osmotic laxatives** and **stimulant laxatives**. Osmotic medications work by drawing water into the colon, which helps keep stool soft and speeds up transit time through the colon. Examples include MiraLAX (polyethylene glycol) and all forms of magnesium in doses over 350 mg taken all at once. Phillips' Milk of Magnesia, for example, is a form of magnesium called magnesium hydroxide and marketed as an over-the-counter drug, though many people simply buy regular magnesium in the vitamin and mineral aisle and experiment with finding a dose that delivers results. In my practice, I will usually start in the 400 to 600 mg range and bump it up by 200 mg at a time until we identify a helpful and well-tolerated dose, though because I am a nutritionist and not a doctor, I will max out at 1,000 to 1,200 mg and check with a medical doctor before giving the green light to go beyond that dose. These products can take many hours to kick in, so I typically advise dosing them at night to help you move your bowels in the morning, or taking them in the morning if you are among the rarer breed of night poopers. MiraLAX is a safer option than magnesium for people with kidney disease. Osmotic laxatives are typically well tolerated; the main side effect people may complain of is bloating (from the water they can draw into the colon) and/or diarrhea when the dose is too high.

Stimulant laxatives work by causing the inner lining of the colon to contract more regularly. Examples include bisacodyl (marketed as Dulcolax) and senna, which can be marketed as a dietary supplement or a tea, or in standardized doses as an over-the-counter medication (Senokot, ex-lax). In the past, these types of medications were used with greater caution for concerns about them being tolerance-forming or damaging the colon (so-called cathartic colon). These concerns related to old-school laxatives that are no longer in circulation, and have not been shown to apply to products currently available. When taken in recommended doses, stimulant laxatives are safe for long-term use. The main tolerance complaint with stimulant laxatives is that some people can find them crampy. Diarrhea can also be an issue. Adjusting the dose down can sometimes mitigate these unpleasant side effects. If you are pregnant, ask your doctor what types of laxatives they prefer for you to use if needed.

Fiber Supplements

Fiber supplements can be hit-or-miss when you have slow transit constipation. They're not my first choice unless I've determined that a person's diet is really lacking in fiber. Oftentimes, someone with slow transit constipation or IBS-C is already somewhat backed up with retained stool such that taking a fiber supplement feels like "adding cars to a traffic jam," to borrow a brilliant analogy from my fellow GI dietitian and author Kate Scarlata.

Some people with IBS-C do find fiber supplements to be helpful, however, so in the spirit of experimenting with bowel regimen, it certainly isn't unreasonable to try out a fiber supplement. As I explained in the previous chapter on fiber imbalance, I tend to recommend more bulking varieties of fiber for my constipated patients, as these have high water-holding capacity. The best-studied and most effective products for constipation include psyllium husk (Metamucil, Konsyl, or its generic forms) and calcium polycarbophil (Fiber-Con). Psyllium is available in powdered form (watch the sugar content—it can be incredibly high in flavored products), pill form, and wafers. If you prefer pills, an effective dose of FiberCon is just two pills, whereas it can take up to five pills of psyllium to achieve a dose that delivers the same benefits. Fiber supplements absolutely must be taken along with a full glass of water to be effective. Some people find that combining fiber supplements with laxatives as part of a comprehensive bowel regimen is a helpful strategy.

While many fiber supplements containing inulin or poly-dextrose are being marketed in convenient and palatable gummy forms, I tend not to recommend these for my constipated patients. As I described in Chapter 4 on IBS-D and Chapter 9 on fiber imbal-ance, inulin can create significant amounts of gas that people with IBS-C are likely to find very distressing. There are also very few studies that have even tested it as a constipation remedy compared with better-studied psyllium and calcium polycarbophil. Fiber-fortified bars and other processed foods that contain inulin, which is also known as chicory root fiber, may have a similar gassy and bloat-ing effect (I'm looking at you, low-carb ice-cream pints!). Polydex-trose has not performed well when tested as a constipation remedy against a placebo.

Stool Softeners and Lubricants

Some over-the-counter medications help manage constipation by softening stools, making them easier to pass, though they are not laxatives per se. Colace (docusate sodium) works by lowering the surface tension of stool, which allows more water to enter into it. It is safe for pregnant and breastfeeding women, and is often given to women after childbirth as well to reduce the need to strain to pass bowel movements. Another option is mineral oil, which is a taste-less, slick, indigestible oil that's taken by mouth and stays within your digestive tract, penetrating and coating stools so they can slip out comfortably and more easily. It's a fine short-term measure if you are going through an especially difficult phase of abnormally hard stools—say, after a vacation when you got extra backed up. I don't typically recommend it as a longer-term solution because it can cause malabsorption of fat-soluble vitamins (vitamins A, D, E, and K) and therefore lead to nutritional deficiencies over time.

Enemas and Suppositories

In extreme cases of slow transit constipation, you may not respond adequately to even a layered regimen of multiple laxatives that work in a complementary way. When this is the case, over-the-counter **enemas** can provide much-needed relief by dislodging some of the stool that's sitting in the rectum—the last six- to eight-inch segment of the colon—and coaxing it out. If you get very lucky, sometimes releasing this bit of stool at the end can even encourage more stool farther upstream to flow out, almost as if a cork has been unplugged. Enemas involve squirting a liquid directly into the rectum, which loosens stool and helps flush it out. There are different types of enemas available. Saline (saltwater) enemas can help draw more water into the bowel like an osmotic laxative would. If you have advanced kidney disease, saline enemas should not be used without explicit approval of your nephrologist (kidney doctor). Stimulant enemas contain bisacodyl, the same medication as in Dulcolax that can stimulate contractions of the inner lining of the colon. Lubricating enemas contain mineral oil and may help hard plugs of stool slide out more easily. Enemas are safe, they start working within minutes, and can be used regularly if needed. A company called Fleet markets the primary brand of enema products in the United States, but there are many store-brand and generic options available.

Similarly, rectal **glycerin suppositories** can be a cheap, safe, fast, and effective way to trigger a bowel movement almost on demand and obtain some relief. These are waxy, bullet-shaped inserts that you put right into your rectum; their presence there can stimulate anal sphincter muscle relaxation and, in turn, the urge and ability to move out some stool that's been waiting on deck. Often, this can have a similar uncorking effect as the enemas described above and coax out a significant amount of stool. Suppositories are less messy than enemas since they don't use any liquid. I find that suppositories are a very underutilized tool in the constipation tool kit, possibly because they're old-fashioned and low-tech. For patients of mine with slow transit constipation or IBS-C, I often recommend using a suppository as a rescue remedy if their usual bowel regimen hasn't produced the expected bowel movement by about 10 a.m., when many people's window of poop-ortunity is closing. This helps ensure you won't skip a day, as skipping can be exceedingly miserable for my patients with IBS-C. Another way I suggest using suppositories is to help trigger a later afternoon or evening bowel movement when needed. Many of my patients really only get the urge to move their bowels earlier in the day—mornings or after lunch at the latest. If they find themselves feeling extremely bloated in the lower abdomen before or after dinner in a manner that suggests a significant amount of stool is in position, but they aren't like to have an urge to defecate until the next morning, a suppository can be a quick-acting intervention that provides the impetus. Fleet also markets a variety of suppositories, though many generic and store-brand products are available.

Prescription Medications

There are two main categories of prescription medications used to treat slow transit constipation and IBS-C. **Secretagogues** are medications that act by increasing secretions by the cells that line the inner layer of the colon. This softens stools and increases movement within the bowel. Examples include Amitiza (lubiprostone), Linzess (linaclotide), and Trulance (plecanatide). The main differences among these are the mechanisms by which they open and close cellular ion channels to stimulate secretions. The most common side effect of all these medications is diarrhea, which may or may not be manageable by adjusting the dose.

Serotonergic agents are medications that promote motility by activating peristalsis—or waves of muscular contractions—by triggering a specific kind of serotonin receptor in the gut. (See Chapter 4 on IBS-D for a detailed discussion about the role of the hormone serotonin in your gut's motility patterns.) Motegrity (prucalopride) is an example of a medication in this class. Motegrity is unique in that it seems to enhance motility throughout the entire digestive tract, not just the colon, so it can be useful for people with slow small bowel transit as well, including people predisposed to recurrent SIBO (Chapter 6).

Surgery for Constipation

In extreme cases of slow transit constipation called **colonic iner-tia**, the colon's motility may be so impaired and so unresponsive to even aggressive regimens of medications, enemas, and diet change that surgery is considered as a treatment option. Surgeries that remove part or even all the colon, called partial or total **colec-tomy**, are a last resort to address severe constipation that is lead-ing to other health complications or extreme quality-of-life issues. One surgical option involves reconnecting the remaining part of your bowel to the rectum, essentially keeping the overall internal plumbing intact but shortening the journey for waste to exit the body. Another possibility involves routing the remaining bowel outside the body through an opening in the abdomen called an **ostomy**. If you have an ostomy, your waste will exit the body into a bag you wear outside your body called an ostomy bag. This bag can be emptied throughout the day into a toilet and changed when needed. Once the surgical site has healed, you may be a candi-date for a second surgery in which doctors will reconnect the small intestine back to the rectum. This will enable you to have bowel movements in the typical anatomical manner. When this type of surgery is successful, you may find yourself needing to move your bowels four to six times per day, though it's not uncommon to have to go more often than that. If you are considering a surgical solu-tion, I encourage you to consult with a colorectal surgeon who is experienced with motility disorders.

Dietary Approaches for Managing IBS-C and Slow Transit Constipation

Irritable bowels do best when they have a consistent, predictable routine, and diet is very much integral to the routine when it comes to managing constipation.

Establish a Consistent Morning Routine, Including Coffee and Breakfast

Morning is the time of day that our bowels are primed to poop due to high circulating levels of the bowel-rousing hormone cortisol. If you are also employing a bedtime bowel regimen—perhaps an osmotic laxative and/or some supplemental fiber—then morning is your optimal window of poop-ortunity, and you'll want conditions to be perfect to make the magic happen.

I'd recommend you aim to wake up early enough to allow for coffee and breakfast before 10 a.m., after which time cortisol levels naturally start to decline. Coffee has a natural compound called **chlorogenic acid** that stimulates the colon, so if you don't drink it, you're missing out on an opportunity to pile onto the strong motility signal we're trying to send to your bowels. If caffeine makes you jittery or interferes with your sleep, then decaf coffee will work just fine, too. Remember—it's not the caffeine in coffee that makes it effective, it's the chlorogenic acid. Tea does not have the same effect, nor does hot water with lemon, though it's not uncommon for the very act of eating or drinking *anything* in the morning to help stimulate an urge to defecate.

Eating breakfast is another thing you can do to send a motility message to your colon at this opportune time of day. The act of eating—and of eating something reasonably substantial—triggers a digestive nerve reflex called the **gastrocolic reflex**, which I described in Chapter 2. This reflex involves a nerve signal from the upstream part of the digestive tract (stomach, small intestine) to the downstream part of the digestive tract (colon) that urges it to contract and move its contents forward so as to make room for the incoming meal. When we add up (1) your naturally high morning-cortisol levels with (2) the impact of the laxative or bowel regimen you used the night before with (3) the colon-stimulating effect of coffee and (4) the motility-promoting gastrocolic reflex, your body is about as primed to poop as it's going to be for the rest of the day. Conditions are perfect.

Eat Fewer, Larger Meals Instead of
Small Frequent Meals (If This Is Well Tolerated)

As the previous section's explanation of the gastrocolic reflex implies, people with sluggish motility may find that eating fewer, more consolidated meals—more foods at once, less often—can stimulate their bowels more effectively than grazing on mini meals and snacks throughout the day. The gastrocolic reflex is why we are more likely to have the urge to move our bowels soon after eating a meal, and it may not be triggered enough if you're skipping (or skimping) on breakfast and snacking your way through the afternoon rather than stopping to consume a more substantial meal all at once. This is because larger volumes of food that produce a more pronounced stretch of the stomach's walls, as well as dietary fat, are particularly effective triggers of the gastrocolic reflex. Be advised that large volume doesn't necessarily mean high calorie—a large salad or sizable bowl of brothy soup can be voluminous enough to stimulate the gastrocolic reflex.

Consolidating meals can be a particularly helpful trick so long as eating more in one sitting doesn't cause you pain. A subset of my patients with IBS-C do find that their abdominal pain can kick up after eating larger amounts. For some, taking a dose of **enteric-coated peppermint oil**—like Atrantil, IBgard, or Heather's Tummy Tamers—about an hour before eating can take the edge off. However, if this is not the case for you, then it's OK to skip this piece of advice and stick to smaller meals that don't provoke post-meal pain.

Include Constipation-Countering Superfoods
in Your Regular Diet

Are there foods that are particularly helpful for constipation? Yes! One of them is kiwifruit. There have been a bunch of smaller studies in people with IBS-C or chronic constipation that have found two kiwis per day to improve defecation frequency and/or stool form compared with a placebo, or as effectively as other well-studied constipation remedies like psyllium fiber or prunes. The benefit of kiwi seems to derive from characteristics beyond its fiber content alone and is well tolerated even among people with IBS. Fruits (and fruit juices) that are concentrated sources of fructose and/or sorbitol, poorly absorbed sugars that have an osmotic (water-attracting) effect in the bowel, have also been found to be helpful as constipation remedies. These include mango, figs, and prunes. These fruits are likely to be beneficial whether consumed fresh or dried; prune juice is also helpful for some. If you have IBS-C and are particularly sensitive to gas pain or bloating, use these fruits sparingly until you've determined you can tolerate them comfortably.

Ground flaxseed, also marketed as flaxmeal or linseed, has also shown promise as a constipation remedy in the research literature, and my clinical experience confirms its utility for many people with constipation. I typically recommend one to two tablespoons per day, mixed into oatmeal, smoothies, yogurt, soup, or other moisture-rich foods. (Ground flaxseed absorbs water well and has a bit of a bulking effect, so it should be taken with liquids and/or water-containing meals.) I happen also to like baking with flaxmeal, and occasionally I use it in place of eggs in cookie recipes: To replace one egg, just combine 1 TBSP ground flaxseed with 2½ TBSP water and let the mixture sit for about ten minutes until it's thick and gooey. Flaxseed oil, however, does not contain fiber, and therefore does not have any special laxative properties beyond the general effect that fat can have on stimulating the bowel.

Constipation by Outlet Dysfunction

Pelvic Floor Dysfunction

WE TYPICALLY THINK OF CONSTIPATION as a problem with slowness that may be worsened by a lack of fiber. The most commonly dispensed advice for constipation is therefore based on this assumption: If the colon's motility is lagging and its takes abnormally long for waste to make its way out, then laxatives and/or added fiber are likely to help speed things up. But there are a substantial number of chronically constipated people who don't respond to laxatives sufficiently—or at all—and for whom eating more fiber seems to make things worse, not better. In some cases, this chronic constipation can be accompanied by occasional difficulty with holding in the stool (**fecal incontinence**). These cases often represent a fairly common but widely overlooked cause of constipation: pelvic floor dysfunction (PFD).

Pelvic Floor Dysfunction

The muscles that make up the so-called **pelvic floor** play a role in defecation (pooping), urination, and sexual function. The coccygeus muscle and the levator ani (which itself is actually composed

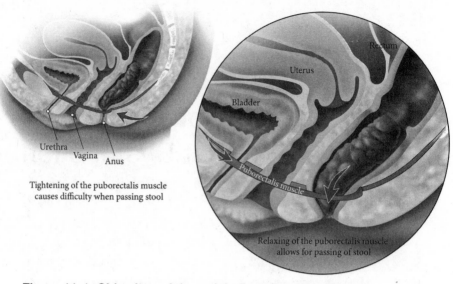

Figure 11-1: Side view of the pelvic floor (person with a uterus/vagina) *Artwork by Mehtonen Medical Studios*

of three separate muscles, including the sling-like puborectalis muscle) are in charge of supporting the rectum, bladder, prostate, or the uterus and vagina (depending on which you were born with). Also in the pelvic floor is the anal sphincter, actually two round muscles that surround and control the opening and closing of the anus (which you may know as the butthole). These sphincter muscles play an important gatekeeper role by contracting (to hold stool in) or relaxing (to allow passage of stool). If the anal sphincters are not working properly, there can also be problems with defecation. The term "pelvic floor dysfunction" refers to a variety of scenarios in which one or more of the pelvic floor muscles is not working properly, and it can result in constipation, as well as other problems, including urinary issues like frequency or urinary incontinence (not being able to hold in pee), chronic prostatitis, fecal incontinence (not always being able to hold in stool), and/or painful vaginal sexual intercourse.

Pelvic floor dysfunction is surprisingly common, especially considering so few of us have ever even heard of it. It is much more prevalent in people assigned female at birth than in people assigned male at birth—and this is particularly so for cisgender women over the age of forty and people who have given birth. Younger people with a history of anxiety, depression, and/or restrictive eating disorders, though, may also be particularly prone to PFD. In the general population, PFD is thought to affect about 17% of cisgender women and 5% of cisgender men; among people with chronic constipation, research suggests that PFD may be at the root of a whopping 40% of cases! Many of my gastroenterologist colleagues who specialize in managing constipation suspect that these figures are significant underestimates.

There are several types of PFD that result in chronic constipation that fall under the category of **dyssynergic defecation** (also called **anismus** or **pelvic floor dyssynergia**). In this scenario, there is an abnormal coordination of the muscles that play a role in evacuating stool, and the result is a partial obstruction (or blockage) of the stool's passage. For example, the particular sling-shaped muscle called the puborectalis that's supposed to *relax* to allow you to empty your bowels easily may paradoxically *contract*—or tighten/clench—when you sit on the toilet and attempt to move your bowels. This has the result of *inhibiting* the passage of stool when you sit down on the toilet to go—sort of like creating a kink in the rectum that should be a straight passageway out of the body. The result may be a chronic feeling of incomplete emptying, needing to strain even when the stool's texture is soft, having very infrequent bowel movements (fewer than three per week), and/or inadequate response to laxative medications. See the inset illustration in Figure 11-1, which represents this phenomenon. Beyond dyssynergia, there are other types of pelvic muscle dysfunction that can affect your ability to move your bowels effectively as well; these include certain muscles that are too tight, certain muscles that are too weak, and diminished sensation in your rectum when there's stool present there that's ready to be eliminated.

When you cannot pass complete stools on a chronic basis, your colon will start to back up with more and more retained stool. The result is what we call a high **stool burden**—a stool backlog as I often like to call it. When your colon is full of stool in this manner, it can often be seen or felt by a trained gastroenterologist examining your abdomen. A colon full of stool can also be visualized on X-ray or via other imaging methods, such as ultrasound or CT scan. People who struggle with pelvic floor dysfunction may have particular stool buildup in the left side of their colon. Symptom-wise, you may experience bloating and visible distension that is worse as the day progresses with each additional meal, sharp or crampy abdominal pain after larger meals, and/or significant amounts of fecal-smelling flatulence toward the end of the day no matter what foods you've eaten (or what foods you've excluded). Some of my patients can even experience upper digestive symptoms, like nausea or early fullness from meals, when their stool burden is particularly high. Many of my backed-up patients with PFD often comment that they feel their best when they eat "unhealthy" foods—by which they mean low-fiber things like pasta or a sandwich—and their worst when they eat the healthiest—by which they typically mean high-fiber foods like salads.

Diagnosing PFD

Digital Rectal Exam

If your gastroenterologist suspects PFD, they may conduct a variety of assessments. A **digital rectal exam**, in which they insert a gloved, lubricated finger into your rectum while you attempt to relax and squeeze your anal muscles—as well as bear down (push)—is one such assessment method. Your doctor's perception of the tightness and weakness of these basic anorectal muscle functions may suggest the need for further testing.

Anorectal Manometry

A more objective way to assess the functioning of pelvic floor muscles is a test called **anorectal manometry**, which is conducted in a specialist gastroenterologist's office and takes only about ten to fifteen minutes. After prepping for the test with an at-home enema, you will have a thin tube with a balloon attached inserted into your rectum. You will perform squeezing and pushing maneuvers, and the catheter balloon will be inflated to test your reflexes and conscious sensation. You will also try to expel the balloon as if it were a stool. The machine's sensors will measure the pressure of the muscles associated with defecation and provide other types of data that will help diagnose many functional issues that could be contributory to your constipation issues. The data allow a skilled gastroenterologist to differentiate between different types of pelvic floor dysfunction so that a proper treatment can be tailored to your individual problem.

MR Defecography

Another diagnostic method for PFD is called **MR defecography**; it is done at a radiologist's office using MRI technology to visualize the pelvic floor muscles in action as they attempt to pass a contrast substance inserted into your rectum via enema. By watching the pooping muscles in real time, doctors can see whether they are coordinating properly. This test also allows doctors to diagnose the presence of a structural defect called a **rectocele** that can affect people with vaginas. A rectocele is a bulge in the muscular back wall of the vagina that separates it from the rectum. This bulge is caused by muscle weakness and creates a pocket where stool can get lodged on its way out, making it difficult to completely empty. Often, people who suffer from constipation related to a rectocele will instinctively learn to press down on their perineum (the pad of flesh between the anus and the genitals) or insert a finger into their vagina and push up against the back wall in order to help them complete bowel movements. This latter technique is called **vaginal splinting**.

Treating PFD

Pelvic floor dysfunction is typically more responsive to medical interventions than diet change, and the nature of the medical intervention will vary based on the type of pelvic floor dysfunction you have. The gold standard for treating dyssynergic defecation is physical therapy that includes **biofeedback therapy**, a type of nerve and muscle retraining administered by a specialized pelvic floor physical therapist that helps improve sensory perception and muscle coordination in the anal sphincter and rectum. It's the gold standard for very good reason: Biofeedback has a high success rate! Research suggests that 70% to 80% of patients with dyssynergic defecation experience substantial symptom improvement following a relatively brief course of biofeedback therapy. Even better: another study followed up with success stories two years after completing treatment and found that 80% of them reported that their improvements persisted.

Biofeedback may involve guided exercises during an internal vaginal or rectal exam or using electromyography (electrodes attached to your body that measure activity of muscles); using visual or audio aids to help you observe how your pelvic floor muscles react when you attempt to contract and relax; practicing expelling a balloon inserted into your rectum via a catheter; and/or practicing toileting techniques to help prevent clenching and straining when sitting down to go, including breathing methods and positioning modifications. As you practice the guided exercises during a treatment session, the therapist or the biofeedback machine will signal when the muscles have coordinated properly so you can practice the mechanics over and over until they become under your conscious control.

Biofeedback therapy sessions are typically administered every one to two weeks for six sessions or so, whereas pelvic floor physical therapy may occur once or twice weekly for at least six to eight weeks, and in complex cases it can require many months of treatment. A pelvic floor physical therapist will also likely teach you about **diaphragmatic breathing techniques** during defecation and optimal **toileting positions** that help ensure your abdominal and pelvic floor muscles are relaxed and aligned to allow for perfect poo passage. Placing a step stool in front of your toilet is a key recommendation to ensure proper toileting position, as it allows your knees to be elevated above your hips to mimic the squatting position that best promotes stool passage.

Beyond biofeedback, there are other medical treatments doctors may use to treat other types of pelvic floor problems. Issues with anal muscle function may be treated with injections of botulinum toxin (Botox) to help relax too-tight sphincter muscles, though prescription **rectal or vaginal suppositories** that contain muscle-relaxing medications like Valium or baclofen may also be an option for some. **Pelvic floor physical therapy** (without biofeedback) that involves strengthening or muscle coordination may also be indicated. Any or all these therapies might also be combined with a regimen of laxatives and/or fiber supplements to complement the work, but treatment regimens should be tailored to your individual issues. For example, while supplemental fiber may improve defecation completeness in someone with a rectocele, it may aggravate symptoms in someone with untreated dyssynergic defecation who is already carrying a high stool burden.

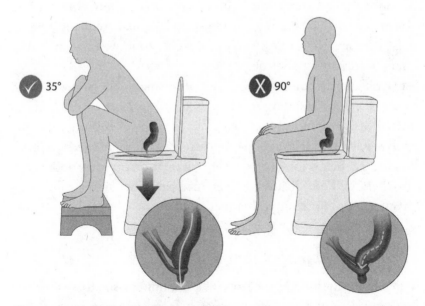

Figure 11-2: Optimal toileting position *Artwork by Mehtonen Medical Studios*

While laxatives aren't a silver bullet fix for people with pelvic floor dysfunction, there are still some remedies that can offer partial relief of constipation—especially as a temporary measure until proper diagnosis and treatment can be completed. Some people find that over-the-counter laxatives can stimulate more frequent urges to defecate—and in many cases, **stimulant laxatives** like senna (marketed as Senokot or ex-lax) or bisacodyl (marketed as Dulcolax) may be more effective than **osmotic laxatives** like magnesium (marketed as Phillips' Milk of Magnesia) or polyethylene glycol 3350 (marketed as MiraLAX). Your doctor may also offer you a prescription laxative option as well. If medication is not effective at all, you may find that remedies inserted directly into the rectum have a higher success rate at coaxing out some stool, probably because they largely bypass the problematic segment of the pelvic floor. Examples include rectal **glycerin suppositories** or **enemas**—both widely available over-the-counter options. These can help you release at least some stool on a regular basis to relieve the severity of your bloating and discomfort until a longer-term treatment can be worked out. Glycerin suppositories are waxy little bullets that you insert into your rectum. Their presence in the rectum can stimulate anal sphincter muscle relaxation and, in turn, the urge and ability to move out some stool that's been waiting on deck.

Collectively, the combination of medications, suppositories, enemas, and/or toileting techniques you use on a regular basis to help move your bowels is referred to as a **bowel regimen**. People with pelvic floor dysfunction often rely on a multipronged approach to manage their symptoms—some combination of pelvic floor physical therapy/biofeedback, laxatives, medical interventions, fiber supplements, and toileting techniques.

Dietary Management of PFD

Pelvic floor dysfunction is more of a plumbing issue than a dietary one, so medical interventions that help correct the muscle dysfunction are going to make much more of an impact on symptoms than diet change. But while diet can't cure PFD, there are certainly some dietary patterns that can exacerbate the bloating and discomfort associated with constipation from PFD that has not yet been treated. As such, the role of diet in suspected or untreated PFD is to reduce the severity of the constipation and its related symptoms. This typically comes down to how you approach the fiber in your diet—namely, how much of it you consume and in what form.

When the pelvic floor muscles cannot effectively pass complete stools and you are already retaining a significant amount of backed-up stool, loading up on a high-fiber diet may actually make you feel worse, not better. I tailor my approach with patients to how backed up they seem to be, and how much stool they are able to pass on a daily basis with the aid of a bowel regimen (see the discussion above). People who are able to move a reasonable amount of stool on a daily or every-other-day basis may have more latitude with how much fiber they can consume comfortably compared with people who can only move their bowels once or twice per week. Relatedly, people who can pass larger, bulkier, more complete stools on their bowel regimen may tolerate more fiber than people who can only pass hard little balls of stool. As I constantly remind my patients: All fiber that goes in must eventually come out. If your bowel regimen does not yet enable you to pass a significant amount *out* each day, you're not going to feel good putting a significant amount *in* each day. If you follow an extremely high-fiber diet, it is often helpful to try pulling back on the amount of fiber you consume by about 25% to 30% as a starting point, and then figuring out if you need to adjust further based on how you feel. After all, as I shared in Chapter 10, my dietitian colleague Kate Scarlata quips that eating loads of fiber when you are already totally full of stool is like "adding cars to a traffic jam." Putting more cars on the road doesn't make the traffic move any quicker when there's total gridlock at the intersection.

Regardless of the amount of fiber that feels best for you, I typically steer my patients with PFD away from bulky types of **insoluble fiber** that take up a lot of real estate in the already-full colon. Softer, mushier, shape-shifting forms of **soluble fiber** (see Chapters

4 and 12)—as well as any fiber-rich foods that have been mechanically altered in a blender or food processor to minimize the particle size of the fiber—are often best tolerated among people who are
already quite full of stool. As I described in the beginning of Chapter 9 (page 196), insoluble fiber is the type of fiber found in leafy
vegetables, fruit and vegetable skins, whole wheat/wheat bran, seeds,
and nuts. Chapter 12 describes a moderate-fiber, gentle-fiber dietary
pattern that may be most suitable for people with PFD who have a
hard time emptying their bowels completely, and Table 7-1 on page
145 in the chapter on inflammatory bowel disease also offers some
ideas on texture modification of fiber-containing foods.

Case Study: Martin's Ulcerative Colitis with a Side of Pelvic Floor Dysfunction

Martin was first referred to me for dietary management of his ulcerative colitis and proctitis (autoimmune inflammation of both the
colon and rectum; Chapter 7), and he was in the middle of a very
active flare at the time. He was a health-conscious, weekend-warrior
type who ate a healthy diet and loved to cycle long distances on
the weekends. During an active colitis flare-up, he suffered from
diarrhea and constant, sometimes unproductive, urges to move his
bowels. But even when his colitis was in remission, he complained
of constant feelings of lower-abdominal pressure and some post-
meal pain in the upper-left quadrant of his abdomen. On these days,
he would wake feeling bloated, have a normal-formed bowel movement in the morning, which temporarily alleviated his bloating, but
then his symptoms of bloating, pressure, and pain would build as the
day progressed.

A detailed diet history revealed that Martin's healthy diet was
not just high in fiber but was extremely high in insoluble fiber—
the "roughage" type of fiber that adds bulk to stool and does a lousy
job holding on to moisture. As he recounted high-fiber meal after
high-fiber meal to me, it became pretty clear that one single normal bowel movement was not going to be nearly enough stool output to keep pace with the amount of fiber Martin was consuming. I

recommended a gentle fiber diet (page 252) to help align the amount of fiber he was consuming with the amount of stool he seemed able to pass each morning, and to reduce the bulky textured fiber I suspected was causing him pain in the setting of being backed up.

I didn't see Martin again for a full year. He came back reporting that he had adopted the diet changes I recommended and they'd helped a lot for about six months, but slowly some of his symptoms started creeping back. On his lower-fiber, gentle-textured diet, the bloating was gone, but he was still struggling with that lower-abdominal pressure and occasional post-meal pain that he now recognized as a function of being constipated, even though he was having a bowel movement each day. His doctor had recently ordered an X-ray and told Martin that his bowels were completely full of stool, even though Martin had gone twice that morning before the X-ray was taken! Not knowing what to do following the X-ray results, he'd put himself on a **stool softener**, started using senna as a laxative a few times per week, and made an appointment to see me.

Between Martin's history of chronic diarrhea (requiring him to reflexively "hold it in" a lot) and his passion for cycling (a sport that puts a lot of pressure on the pudendal nerve that plays a role in proper pelvic floor function for urination, sexual function, and defecation), I began to wonder whether he might have developed some type of pelvic floor dysfunction along the way that was preventing him from being able to empty his bowels completely. I suggested the possibility to Martin's gastroenterologist, who referred him for an anorectal manometry test. The manometry confirmed a diagnosis of pelvic floor dyssynergia: One of Martin's pelvic floor muscles was paradoxically contracting when it was supposed to be relaxing as he sat down to defecate, and this had the effect of choking off the flow of stool out of the rectum. The test also showed that Martin's anal sphincter remained slightly too tight during the act of defecation, which had an effect akin to trying to squeeze toothpaste out of a tube whose opening is half-blocked.

After eight weeks of pelvic floor physical therapy with biofeedback, Martin was reporting far greater ease with defecation and he was passing more stool volume on a day-to-day basis. Still, about two or three times per month, he'd experience what he described as a spasm that had him running to the bathroom thinking he needed to defecate, only to find there was nothing but gas or the teensiest bit of stool. His doctor prescribed a Valium rectal suppository for use on these occasions to relax the anal sphincter muscles and stop the spasm and sent him back for another month of physical therapy just to be sure the work was finished.

I saw Martin again two years later when he was seeking dietary advice for a completely different issue—not gastrointestinal related. Digestively, he told me, he'd been doing so incredibly well! He was following the gentle fiber diet about 75% of the time and taking stool softeners each night, and by doing so he'd been able to comfortably reintroduce salads for lunch about three times per week. Now that his pelvic floor muscle coordination was working properly, he was not at risk for becoming extremely backed up again when fiber intake was a bit higher. He still kept the Valium suppositories on hand for as-needed use, though episodes of spasms only happened a few times per year, often when he was traveling or otherwise off his usual diet and exercise routine. Martin's case was a true success story that speaks to the potential for significant and durable progress from targeted treatments for a well-defined pelvic floor problem.

PART IV

Dietary Remedies to Restore Regularity

Fiber-Modified Diets for Both Diarrhea and Constipation

AS I DESCRIBED IN THE introduction of Chapter 9 (page 195), fiber refers to plant-based carbohydrates that humans cannot digest and absorb. Because the fiber we eat does not ever leave the gut, it plays a key role in regulating our bowel movements. The amount and type of fiber we eat affects the size and consistency of our stools, and it also influences how quickly stool moves through the colon— our digestive transit time. For these reasons, one of the primary ways you can regulate your bowel movements is by modifying the amount and type of fiber you consume. This chapter will describe some of the common ways I manipulate dietary fiber or use fiber supplements to help manage irregular bowel movements in the various patient populations I work with.

Soluble Fiber Therapy

Best for:

- Diarrhea-predominant IBS (IBS-D)

- Diarrhea due to rapid transit (after a bowel resection surgery, for example)

- Mild ulcerative colitis or Crohn's disease

Soluble fiber therapy is an intervention I use to help patients with diarrhea from a variety of origins, and it's long been among the most effective tricks I have up my sleeve. It refers to changing your diet and/or using supplements to increase your intake of a particular type of fiber called soluble fiber—which has a water-absorbing, transit-time-slowing, poo-consolidating effect in the colon. Simultaneously, you will reduce your intake of insoluble fiber—the colon-stimulating, speed-inducing roughage that isn't able to hold on to much moisture as it passes through the digestive tract. The result? Soft but formed, less urgent, longer, and fuller poops that leave you feeling more completely evacuated with fewer trips to the bathroom. (Kind of sounds like a dream, doesn't it?) If you need a refresher on soluble and insoluble fiber, flip back to Chapter 9 on page 195.

Who Benefits Most from Soluble Fiber Therapy?

Soluble fiber therapy works best for people with diarrhea caused by rapid transit through the intestines or attacks of spasm-like colon contractions—such as in the case of diarrhea-predominant irritable bowel syndrome (IBS-D). People who may suffer from watery, urgent, too-frequent, or too-loose stools from rapid transit also include those who have had intestinal surgeries that resulted in a shorter-than-normal bowel, whether due to inflammatory bowel disease, diverticular disease, colorectal cancer, bowel injuries or obstructions, or severe motility problems like colonic inertia. People with short bowel syndrome (SBS) who have only one-third or less of their small intestine remaining often benefit from one or more supplemental doses of soluble fiber each day to help prevent **dehydration** and malnutrition by slowing down intestinal contents long enough to be absorbed into the body.

Fiber supplements are almost universally marketed as remedies for constipation, but in my clinical practice, I am far more likely to recommend them to help manage diarrhea, frequent bowel movements, or urgent bowel movements. It seems counterintuitive to my diarrhea-prone patients that I advise them to try out a fiber supplement—and downright scary to my patients who suffer from severe diarrhea and even fecal incontinence who worry that more fiber will only make things worse. In some cases, patients express worry that a fiber supplement will work too well and actually constipate them! But for most of my patients with IBS-D, it only takes a few days before they're convinced. This stuff is one of the most effective remedies for many types of diarrhea that stem from rapid transit or similar motility issues; it's safe, it's widely available, and it's not expensive.

If your bowels are most active in the morning, then I typically recommend taking a soluble fiber supplement at some point in the evening, because it takes many hours for the fiber to travel to the colon where it works its magic. If you are diarrhea prone during the day, try dosing the fiber in the morning. Many of my patients with shorter guts as a result of prior surgeries find it helpful to take a few half doses or full doses over the course of a day. In truth, dosing fiber supplements is as much art as it is science, and often we need to experiment a bit with different doses and times until we land on the perfect bowel regimen. Regardless of what you take and when, however, it's important to take a fiber supplement with a full (8 oz.) glass of water or other liquid. As I shared in Chapter 9, my gastroenterologist colleague Dr. Eric Goldstein warns his patients that they may "make bricks, not poops" if they supplement fiber without co-ingesting adequate water.

Table 12-1: How to Use Soluble Fiber Supplements to Manage Irregularity

Product/Ingredient	Dosing	Most Likely to Benefit
Methylcellulose (marketed as Citrucel)	2 g fiber/serving in a standard dose, which is equivalent to 1 TBSP Citrucel powder or 4 tablets, taken with 8 oz. water Take in the evening/bedtime to address problematic morning bowel movements	People with diarrhea-predominant irritable bowel syndrome (IBS-D) who experience multiple, urgent, loose bowel movements in the morning
Wheat dextrin (active ingredient in the US version of Benefiber) The Canadian version contains a different active ingredient called inulin, which I do not recommend for managing irregular bowel patterns.	2 g fiber/serving in a standard dose of 2 tsp. powder to be mixed in 8 oz. water This product comes in powder form only; it is flavorless and colorless and not gritty	People with diarrhea-predominant irritable bowel syndrome (IBS-D) who experience multiple, urgent, loose bowel movements in the morning Not appropriate for people with celiac disease (product is wheat-derived)
Partially hydrolyzed guar gum, or PHGG (marketed as Benefiber Advanced Digestive Health, Regular Girl, Sunfiber)	4–5 g fiber/1 TBSP serving of powder in most products	People with diarrhea-predominant irritable bowel syndrome (IBS-D) who experience multiple, urgent, loose bowel movements in the morning
Acacia fiber (marketed as Heather's Tummy Fiber or generic)	4 g fiber/2 tsp. serving of powder in most products Start with a 1 tsp. dose and increase to 2 tsp. per dose, or add a second daily 1 tsp. dose as needed/beneficial	People with diarrhea-predominant irritable bowel syndrome (IBS-D) who experience multiple, urgent, loose bowel movements in the morning

Table 12-1 *(continued)*

Product/Ingredient	Dosing	Most Likely to Benefit
Psyllium husk (marketed as Konsyl, Metamucil, or generic; may also be known as ispaghula)	3–6 g of fiber is a therapeutic dose; this is equivalent to 1–2 tsp. of powder (read the product's label) Psyllium is available in capsules, but due to its bulk, you may need to consume up to five capsules to achieve the therapeutic dose	People with mixed-type IBS who are prone to both constipation AND diarrhea Some surgeons recommend it following a bowel surgery to help bulk up stools and prevent both diarrhea and constipation Psyllium supplements have also been shown to help lower cholesterol
Calcium polycarbophil* (marketed as FiberCon)	1 g of calcium polycarbophil in a standard dose of two capsules (FiberCon; 500 mg each). Take with 8 oz. water (or fluid) per dose Can increase by one pill at a time, with adequate water as needed	People with watery diarrhea or fecal incontinence (accidents) due to very rapid transit or a shorter bowel (e.g., after an intestinal surgery) or due to weak anal or rectal muscle function Also people with IBS-C (constipation-predominant IBS) who have infrequent, incomplete stools; it often works even better when used alongside a laxative

* While calcium polycarbophil is not technically a soluble fiber, it behaves very similar to one in terms of its bulking and water-holding properties. This synthetic compound has the ability to absorb a substantial amount of water and is one of the heavier-duty remedies available to address severe watery diarrhea due to rapid transit. This product has been used successfully in many patients who suffered from fecal incontinence (pooping accidents) following intestinal surgeries or resections; after all, a very bulky, formed stool is far less likely to slip out accidentally than a watery, loose one!

You'll notice that the table above does not include any fiber gummy product recommendations. This is because the sources of fiber used in fiber gummies—typically inulin, chicory, or polydextrose—do not have great data on their efficacy for regulating bowel movements. What's more is that many people find inulin to be extremely gassy; see Chapter 4, page 72, for a more detailed discussion on inulin and why I shy away from recommending it for my digestively distressed patients.

My patients with IBS-D who have suffered for years routinely use the term "life-changing" to describe the effect of a single dose of soluble fiber taken in the evening. For many, it can truly be that effective. If you're someone used to spending the entire morning every morning running back and forth to the bathroom four, five, or six times until your overactive colon is done emptying itself in fits of crampy urgency, soluble fiber therapy can often transform your chaotic morning toileting routine into a calmer, predictable pattern of one or two larger, more formed, complete bowel movements that enable you to get out of the house far earlier.

I have also been known to successfully deploy soluble fiber–rich diets (generally without the supplements) for my patients with constipation due to constipation-predominant IBS. If you're someone who is able to move your bowels a little tiny bit each day but never feel completely evacuated, with stools that are typically hard little balls despite a high-fiber diet, or you experience crampy abdominal pain after eating large salads, you may have the type of constipation that responds well to a soluble fiber–rich diet, too.

So how does it work? Soluble fiber slows down intestinal transit time. Not in a constipating way, mind you: It's still fiber, and it contributes to a bulky stool that eases defecation. Rather, it has a regulating effect that helps you find a happy middle ground between diarrhea and constipation. (If only it would run for Congress!) It's named for the fact that it's water-soluble, or it dissolves in water, forming a gel-like, viscous, gooey, gummy consistency; for a mental image, picture what happens to oats when you leave them to soak in water, or to chia seeds when mixed with milk to form chia pudding. Now picture this sticky, viscous mass making its way through your intestines, sopping up extra water along the way like a sponge until it finally arrives (in its own sweet time) to your colon, adding moist bulk to the rest of the waste and gluing it all together so it can be eliminated efficiently in one fell poop. Your irritable colon can try as it may to spasm and rush it along, but viscous liquids have friction enough to resist rapid flow. And that viscous mass of stool is now quite capable of mounting a resistance to the forces of nature that try to hurry it out.

For people who are constipated, having ample soluble fiber in the diet can help ensure that stools don't get so hard and dried out that they're impossible to pass. Because one of the colon's jobs is to reabsorb water from the waste stream back into the body, stools that spend too much time there may lose too much of their water. This can result in those hard "rabbit pellet"–type poops that are really hard to expel, and leave you feeling incompletely emptied. If you're trying to eat a high-fiber diet to help with your constipation—but the primary fiber in your diet comes from insoluble sources like lettuce and salads, nuts, berries, popcorn, and whole wheat products—you may find that there's not enough soluble fiber in the waste stream to hold on to moisture for the slow journey. In these cases, changing the balance of fiber in your diet to skew more toward soluble fiber sources can help tremendously. See Table 12-2 below for a list of soluble fiber–rich foods toward which you may consider distorting your intake.

Table 12-2: Soluble Fiber–Rich Foods

Fruits	Apples (peeled)
	Apricots
	Avocados
	Bananas and plantains
	Clementines, mandarins, oranges, tangerines
	Mangoes
	Melons
	Nectarines
	Papaya
	Peaches
	Pears
Vegetables	Asparagus tips
	Beets
	Broccoli florets
	Carrots
	Cauliflower florets
	Chayote squash (peeled)
	Cucumber (peeled)
	Eggplant (peeled)
	Green beans (haricot vert, string beans)
	Jicama (may be gassy in larger quantities)
	Mushrooms
	Okra
	Pumpkin
	Radish
	Rutabaga
	Turnip
	Winter squash (e.g., acorn, butternut, delicata, kabocha [peeled])
	Yams/sweet potatoes (without skin)
	Zucchini (and yellow summer squash)
Grains	Barley
	Oats (and oat bran, oat flour)
Nuts/Seeds	Chestnuts (peeled)
	Chia seeds

A Sample Day on a
Soluble Fiber–Rich Diet

A soluble fiber–rich diet can be adjusted to meet your specific needs; in cases of constipation, your goal is to balance your intake of different types of fibers more evenly between insoluble fiber ("roughage") and soluble fiber, whereas if you tend more toward diarrhea, your goal is to skew your fiber intake more heavily toward soluble sources. For some people this may mean that small, appetizer-size salads are still on the table, but maybe not giant entrée-size ones. For very diarrhea-prone people, though, even small amounts of leafy greens—or other insoluble fiber–rich foods like coleslaw, popcorn, nuts, and seeds—can pose a problem. It usually takes some trial and error to find the balance that works for you.

One strategy that can help improve tolerance of insoluble fiber–predominant foods like leafy greens, nuts, and beans is to puree them: minimizing the particle size of the fiber makes it less bulky as it passes through the digestive tract, and therefore somewhat less stimulating to the colon. Think almond butter instead of almonds, spinach in your smoothie instead of piled on your plate as a side dish, hummus instead of whole chickpeas. Same nutritional value, different digestive impact. For some examples of what a day of soluble fiber–predominant eating might look like, Table 12-3 below offers some healthy inspiration.

Table 12-3: Sample Day on a
Soluble Fiber–Rich or Fiber-Predominant Diet

	Sample Plant-Based Menu	Sample Omnivore Menu	Sample Paleo-Style Menu	Sample Gluten-Free Menu
Breakfast	Oatmeal: Almond butter Chia seeds Cinnamon/maple syrup to taste Nondairy "milk" of your choice Oats Sliced banana	Banana Hard-boiled egg(s) Oat-based breakfast cereal (Cheerios, Life, Oat Bran Flakes, Puffins) Milk of choice	Scrambled eggs Sliced avocado Sliced sweet potatoes	Mango Lassi Smoothie Bowl: ½ cup kefir 1 banana 1 cup frozen mango chunks Blend the kefir with the fresh/frozen fruit and scoop it into a bowl To garnish, sprinkle with: 1 TBSP chia seeds 2 TBSP chopped pistachios Fresh mint leaves Puffed rice cereal
Lunch	Mushroom barley soup Side of avocado toast on multigrain or white bread	Side of baby carrots Tuna or turkey + avocado sandwich on multigrain bread	Grilled chicken breast Riced cauliflower Well-steamed or boiled string beans	Butternut squash or carrot ginger soup Grilled or rotisserie chicken Millet, quinoa, or rice

Table 12-3 *(continued)*

	Sample Plant-Based Menu	Sample Omnivore Menu	Sample Paleo-Style Menu	Sample Gluten-Free Menu
Dinner	Quinoa bowl with: Cooked broccoli florets Peeled/seeded cucumber Roasted sweet potato Sesame oil/soy ginger dressing Shredded carrots Tofu	Beef stew with root vegetables (carrots, onion, potatoes, turnips)	Baked salmon and spiralized zucchini "noodles" tossed with dairy-free pesto Roasted beet/orange salad	Avocado or guacamole Corn tortillas Fat-free refried beans (e.g., Amy's) Ground taco meat Raw chayote squash, peeled and julienned Salsa or pico de gallo + Shredded cheese (optional)
Snack(s) and Treats	Carrots/hummus/tortilla chips Coconut "yogurt" + clementines or orange Health Warrior Chia bar Oatmeal cookie	Beet chips, peeled cucumber spears + tzatziki dipping sauce Bobo's Oat bars or KIND Healthy Grains bar Peeled apple with peanut butter Yogurt of choice or cottage cheese + sliced peaches	Chia Pod (Banana, Blueberry, Mango) or coconut chia pudding Dried apricots Melon Plantain chips with almond butter	Garden Lites Veggie Muffins (frozen section) Nairn's gluten-free oat crackers + jelly/peanut butter Ready-to-eat peeled chestnuts Sliced pear with or without goat cheese spread

Gentle Fiber or GI Gentle Diet

Best for:

- Extreme constipation

- Constipation related to pelvic floor dysfunction

- Moderate to severe inflammatory bowel disease (IBD) with diarrhea

- Inflammatory bowel disease (IBD) with risk of obstructions

Because all fiber is, by definition, indigestible, then all the fiber that goes into the body must come out of the body. But what happens if you struggle with pelvic floor muscle dysfunction or extremely slow transit constipation, and your body is unable to empty an amount of stool that is commensurate with the amount of fiber you eat? The answer is that the excess stool starts building up . . . and up . . . and up . . . and you may wind up with a colon extremely full of stool. As I described in Chapter 11, when you have a colon full of stool and continue to consume a high-fiber diet loaded with bulky forms of fiber like salads, nuts, and fruits with lots of skins, it can be like adding more and more cars to a traffic jam. There's no room on the metaphorical road for all these additional cars, and by piling them on, you're not exactly speeding up traffic ahead.

FOODS TO AVOID OR MODIFY ON A GENTLE FIBER DIET

Whole raw and cooked coarse-textured veggies and leafy greens, such as:

- Beans and lentils
- Broccoli rabe or broccolini (stalks)
- Cabbage

- Collard greens
- Dried fruit
- Escarole
- Fruits/veggies with lots of individual skins:
  - Berries
  - Cherries
  - Corn kernels (canned/frozen corn kernels, corn on the cob, popcorn)
  - Grapes
  - Peas
- Grapefruit membranes (the segmented fruit itself is fine)
- Kale
- Lettuces: endive, iceberg, radicchio, romaine, etc.
- Nuts and seeds (nut butters are OK)
- Raw celery (chopped/cooked such as in soup is OK)
- Skins of thick-skinned fruits and veggies (peeled is OK):
  - Apples
  - Cucumbers
  - Eggplants
  - Potatoes/sweet potatoes
  - Winter squashes (acorn, butternut, delicata, kabocha, pumpkin, etc.)

Note: All items on this list would be OK if pureed, as in a soup or smoothie

---

There are other cases in which eating certain types of fiber—especially bulky, intact forms of insoluble fiber—can aggravate gastrointestinal issues, including a subset of people who have inflammatory bowel diseases like Crohn's disease or ulcerative colitis. During an active flare-up, when the bowel lining is very inflamed, eating significant amounts of bulky fiber can feel like taking a scrub brush to its already-angry, sensitive segments and aggravate pain or diarrhea. Intact forms of tough, bulkier fiber—leafy greens (whether cooked or raw), coarse veggies like cabbage and celery, corn kernels, fruit/veggie/bean skins, leathery dried fruit, nuts, large seeds—can also pose a risk for people who have narrowed sections of the intestines due to inflammation (called stricturing) or scar tissue from prior surgeries. These narrowed segments can act like a bottleneck when a substantial mass of fiber arrives there as a clump and can't make its way through. This may result in a bowel obstruction, which can be a medical emergency.

To avoid these outcomes without having to eliminate all healthy fruits and vegetables completely, we look to modify the physical form of these whole, intact fibers in ways that reduce the particle size of the fiber. While a bowl of coarse, raw kale salad could really pose a problem for someone with inflammatory bowel disease for any of the reasons above, taking that same kale and blending it into a green smoothie would allow you to get all the same nutrients with a far gentler impact on the bowel. Lastly, because all the fiber we eat winds up undigested in the colon, larger amounts of it in any form can stimulate the bowel walls and promote more motility—but more so when the fiber is bulkier and intact. This can be a particular problem if you are already struggling with too-frequent urges to defecate.

What I like to call a **gentle fiber diet**—sometimes referred to as a GI soft, GI gentle, or lower-residue diet—involves (1) limiting your fiber to softer-textured options where the fiber is mushier and more viscous (it can shape-shift, like cooked oatmeal, avocado, or mashed sweet potatoes); and/or (2) mechanically modifying coarser forms of fiber with a blender to reduce the fiber's particle size to take up less physical space, as in a puree or a liquid. It is similar to the soluble fiber–predominant diet described earlier in this chapter, with a few key differences: there is a heavier emphasis on liquid meals and purees to deliver more of the fiber-containing foods in your diet; it's more restrictive with raw vegetables in general, regardless of the fiber type—these are avoided in all but token garnish-size servings; and it's more conservative with the total amount of fiber overall. There are low-fiber versions of this diet for people at risk of obstruction who really need to be extra conservative, and more moderate-fiber versions. My patients often want to pin me down with a precise number of grams of fiber that they should be eating, but the magic number will vary a lot by person. A very general guideline for the moderate-fiber version is about 20 grams per day; a lower-fiber version would be 10 to 15 grams per day. Unless you are using an electronic food diary app that automatically tracks your fiber as you enter your food intake, though, most people find it really hard to keep track of their fiber intake.

A Sample Day on the Gentle Fiber Diet

In addition to soft-textured proteins like eggs or omelets, fish, tofu, chicken, ground meat, and dairy foods, other staples on the gentle fiber diet include avocado, cooked squashes, beets, melon, mango, papaya, banana, fruit smoothies, pureed vegetable or bean soups, nut butters, and hummus. Sushi is a popular choice when taking your gentle fiber diet on the road. Table 7-1 on page 145 in Chapter 7 lists many gentle or small-particle-size forms of fiber that are most suitable on this type of fiber-modified diet, whereas the sidebar earlier in this chapter (page 248) lists high-risk foods that should either be avoided or pureed before eating. Because we are looking to be conservative with the total amount of fiber consumed on a gentle fiber diet, I do not recommend using fiber supplements to manage diarrhea or constipation in most people with the conditions listed as indications for this diet.

Table 12-4: Sample Day on a Gentle Fiber Diet

	Sample Plant-Based Menu	Sample Omnivore Menu	Sample Paleo-Style Menu	Sample Gluten-Free Menu
Breakfast	Smoothie bowl: Puree together ½ cup frozen berries, 3 TBSP nondairy milk of choice, and one sliced frozen banana Serve in a bowl topped with a few TBSP hemp hearts, peanut butter, and puffed rice cereal (for crunch)	Breakfast sandwich: 1–2 slices tomato Avocado Eggs Multigrain or white bread (not whole wheat) Cappucino or latte	Breakfast egg scramble or frittata made with: Breakfast sausages (no casings) Diced/peeled sweet potato Grated/shredded zucchini Nutritional yeast Onions Green juice	Quick cooking or instant certified gluten-free oatmeal (Bob's Red Mill, Glutenfreeda) With or without chocolate hazelnut or hazelnut butter spread stirred in (Justin's, Nutiva) + Cinnamon + Sliced banana
Lunch	Dr. Hilary's or Praeger's brand veggie burger on a regular/not whole-grain bun Topped with avocado or hummus With side of baked sweet potato fries (no skin)	Quesadilla made with cheese, chicken, refried beans, with or without guacamole or Sashimi and sushi with miso soup	Grain-free wrap: Avocado Condiments of choice—mayo, mustard, Paleo, etc. Freshly-sliced roasted turkey (deli counter) Jarred roasted red pepper Siete brand grain-free tortilla wrap + Side of dairy-free tomato soup	Chicken tortilla soup: Crunched-up tortilla chips Hot sauce (optional) Shredded cheese, with or without cubed avocado Shredded chicken Tomato soup base* *If you make from scratch and the recipe calls for corn with or without black beans, just puree them into the soup base before adding chicken and other toppings.

Table 12-4 *(continued)*

	Sample Plant-Based Menu	Sample Omnivore Menu	Sample Paleo-Style Menu	Sample Gluten-Free Menu
Dinner	Chopped onions and zucchini, stirfried with garlic, sesame oil, and soy sauce Teriyaki baked tofu White rice	Beet + goat cheese "salad" (no greens) Pasta Bolognese or spaghetti with meatballs Side of well-cooked green beans	Shrimp fried "rice" made with riced cauliflower: Coconut aminos (instead of sesame oil + soy sauce) Frozen diced carrots Riced cauliflower Scrambled egg Shrimp	Baked salmon Side of (peeled) and roasted white potatoes mixed with roasted butternut squash chunks, seasoned with fresh herbs
Snack(s) and Treats	Coconut yogurt Dark chocolate with peanut butter cups Rice cakes with nut butter Sorbet or vegan ice cream Tortilla chips with guac or hummus	Chewy granola bar Ice cream Rice cake + peanut butter Watermelon Yogurt of choice or cottage cheese + sliced peaches	Baked/peeled apple with cinnamon) Banana topped with almond butter Coconut tapioca pudding (sweeten with honey or maple syrup)	Clementines PopCorners brand chips Tate's gluten-free cookies Yogurt berry smoothie popsicles

Sugar-Restricted Diets

IN CHAPTER 2, WE REVIEWED the digestive process and briefly mentioned the disaccharidase enzymes that help digest various sugars in the small intestine. Then, in Chapter 5, I explained the concept of osmotic diarrhea in great detail, which is what can result when large amounts of these sugars go undigested in the small intestine; see Figure 5-1 on page 83 for a refresher on sugar digestion and absorption. This chapter will provide more specific details about which foods contain which sugars—whether naturally occurring or added—so that if you are experiencing symptoms of a carbohydrate intolerance like lactose intolerance, fructose intolerance, sucrose intolerance, or intolerance to sugar alcohols (polyols), you'll know what foods are safe to eat and what foods to avoid *if you can't use a supplemental digestive enzyme to help you digest them.* If you need a refresher on the various types of carbohydrate intolerances, what causes them, and how they are diagnosed, flip back to Chapter 5, page 81.

You have two options to manage symptoms of a carbohydrate intolerance: Avoid foods that contain the sugar that triggers your symptoms, or use a supplemental enzyme if available to help your body digest and absorb the sugar. If you choose to consume a food you have an intolerance to without using enzymes, you will likely find that your symptoms of gas, bloating, and/or diarrhea will be dose dependent. This is to say that having a small amount of the food or drink with the problematic ingredient in it may provoke only mild symptoms, whereas larger portions may provoke more significant symptoms. These reactions are medically benign, which means that they are not actually harmful for your health. Rather, they can just be very uncomfortable and unpleasant, and can last anywhere from a few hours to a day or so. I, for one, am somewhat lactose intolerant, and yet I sometimes (read: often) choose to eat high-lactose, real ice cream anyway. The consequences of doing so when I stick to a single scoop are minimal, and to me, they're worth putting up with for the pleasure I get from eating ice cream. If I were doubled over in pain from gas, cramps, and diarrhea from eating ice cream in this moderate portion, I'd probably make a greater effort to find a lactose-free alternative *or* carry over-the-counter lactase enzyme supplements with me so I could take them before partaking of ice cream when out and about.

Low-Lactose and Lactose-Free Diet

Best for:

- Lactose intolerance

- Temporary forms of lactose intolerance caused by active celiac disease or Crohn's disease affecting the small intestine

Lactose is milk sugar that occurs naturally in dairy products. It can also be added to sweets, candy, chocolates, and even medications (such as birth control pills) as an inactive filler ingredient. Vegan or plant-based foods will be naturally lactose-free, as will all meats and eggs. Contrary to a pervasive belief, eggs are NOT dairy foods and therefore are naturally lactose-free. Another myth about lactose is that goat and sheep's milk is substantively lower lactose than cow's milk. They aren't, really, but hard, aged cheeses made from all three of these milks should be extremely low in lactose, if not fully lactose-free. This is because as cheese ages longer and longer, the lactose seeps out of the cheese along with the liquid whey. Whey-based cheeses, such as traditionally made ricotta cheese, are therefore extremely high in lactose, as are some whey-based protein supplements.

Lactose intolerance is caused by inadequate production of the digestive enzyme called lactase in your small intestine. Lactase is required to break apart lactose sugar into its two component molecules, glucose and galactose, so they can be absorbed individually. When you consume more lactose sugar than you have the enzyme capacity to digest, the excess lactose goes undigested, unabsorbed, and travels to the colon where it can cause gas, bloating, diarrhea, and/or cramping. The majority of humans are genetically programmed to produce less lactase enzyme as they age, and this will result in some degree of lactose intolerance in many adults. This is called **primary lactose intolerance**. Some people temporarily lose the ability to digest lactose when there has been damage to the lactase enzyme–producing cells of the small intestine. This may happen in inflammatory conditions like uncontrolled celiac disease or active stages of Crohn's disease affecting the small intestine and is called **secondary lactose intolerance**. Typically, secondary lactose intolerance is reversed once healing of the affected segments of small intestine has taken place.

Table 13-1: Low-Lactose Diets for Lactose Intolerance

	High-Lactose Foods (Avoid or Limit or Take Lactase Enzyme Before Consuming)	Moderate-Lactose Foods (Keep Portions Small or Avoid Altogether)	Lactose-Free Foods (Enjoy as Desired)

Beverages and Liquids	A2 Milk
	Bubble tea (Boba tea)
	Buttermilk
	Cappuccinos
	Eggnog
	Horchata
	Hot cocoa (fresh or from a powder mix)
	Lassi drinks
	Lattes
	Milk (cow, goat, sheep)
	Milkshake
	Vietnamese iced coffee
		Dairy-based kefir
		Yogurt-based drinks
			Lactose-free milk
			Nondairy milk substitutes:
			  Almond
			  Cashew
			  Coconut
			  Flax
			  Hemp
			  Oat
			  Pea protein–based
			  Rice

Protein Foods	Cottage cheese Paneer (Indian cottage cheese) Ricotta cheese Whey protein concentrate	Goat and sheep's milk yogurts Greek yogurt Milk protein concentrate Regular yogurt	American cheese Hard/aged cheeses in portions up to 2 oz., such as cheddar, feta, Gruyère, Halloumi, Manchego, Muenster, Parmesan, Swiss, etc. Lactose-free dairy yogurt Mozzarella cheese Nondairy/vegan yogurts made from any of the milk substitutes listed above Queso fresco Whey protein isolate

Table 13-1 *(continued)*

	High-Lactose Foods (Avoid or Limit or Take Lactase Enzyme Before Consuming)	Moderate-Lactose Foods (Keep Portions Small or Avoid Altogether)	Lactose-Free Foods (Enjoy as Desired)
Desserts and Sweets	Anything made with condensed milk or evaporated milk (e.g., key lime pie, some pumpkin pie recipes) Cheesecake Custards, such as crème brûlée, crème caramel, flan, panna cotta Dulce de leche Frozen yogurt Fudge Gelato Ice cream Milk chocolate Milkshakes Mousse Pudding, rice pudding Tres leches cake	Semisweet chocolate Sherbet Whipped cream (large portions)	Cakes, cookies, pastries, pies made with butter but no other dairy/milk ingredients) Lactose-free ice cream Nondairy frozen desserts (ices, plant-based/vegan "ice cream," sorbet)

(continues)

Table 13-1 *(continued)*

	High-Lactose Foods (Avoid or Limit or Take Lactase Enzyme Before Consuming)	Moderate-Lactose Foods (Keep Portions Small or Avoid Altogether)	Lactose-Free Foods (Enjoy as Desired)
Miscellaneous Foods and Ingredients	Dishes made with a bechamel sauce: Cheese sauce–based dishes like homemade macaroni and cheese Moussaka Some lasagnas		Butter Cream cheese Ghee Half-and-half (limit 2 TBSP per serving)

Low-Fructose Diet

Best for:

- Dietary fructose intolerance

Fructose is a naturally occurring sugar present in some fruits, fruit juices and their concentrates, and natural sweeteners like honey and agave nectar. It can also be added to foods and drinks, often sweet condiments and soft drinks, sodas, sports drinks, and energy gels. As a food additive, it may appear on an ingredient list as high-fructose corn syrup (HFCS), crystalline fructose, fructose, or fruit juice concentrate.

Fructose does not require enzymes to digest, and therefore fructose intolerance does not result from an enzyme deficiency. Rather, fructose requires dedicated sugar transporters lining the small intestine to carry it from the bowel into the body. Some people's bodies express more of these transporters than others or have better-functioning transporters than others. Some people express a perfectly normal number of transporters but consume so much fructose in their diets—perhaps from juicing frequently or drinking lots of soda/soft drinks—that they simply overwhelm their bodies' capacity for absorption. Once you max out your individual ability to absorb fructose, whatever you've consumed in excess of your ability to absorb will go undigested and unabsorbed and travel to the colon where it can cause gas, bloating, diarrhea, and/or cramping.

When it comes to dietary management of fructose intolerance, what matters most is how much free fructose a food contains, and how much fructose it contains in excess of another sugar, glucose. When fructose and glucose are consumed in equal balance, the fructose may actually be absorbed by the same pathways as sucrose (table sugar). But when a food contains relatively more fructose than glucose, the potential for fructose malabsorption increases. Table 13-2 contains lists of the foods most and least likely to be tolerated by people with fructose intolerance.

Table 13-2: Low-Fructose Diet for Fructose Intolerance

	High-Fructose Foods (Avoid or Limit or Take Glucose Isomerase Enzyme Before Consuming)	Low-Fructose Foods (Enjoy as Desired)

Beverages and Liquids	Apple juice and cider
	
	Cocktail mixers that contain high-fructose corn syrup (HFCS), such as Bloody Mary mix, ginger ale, grenadine syrup, margarita mixes, Rose's Lime Juice, tonic water
	
	Cranberry juice cocktail and most other fruit juices (including cocktail mixers)
	
	Energy gels/shots, sports drinks made with fructose
	
	Fruit drinks, iced teas, lemonades, or soda made with HFCS
	
	Honey-sweetened drinks (teas, etc.)
	
	Port wines, rum, and sherry
	
	Smoothies made with a juice base or high-fructose fruits, such as green juices made with apple as a base or tomato juice made with HFCS
		100% cranberry juice sweetened with sugar (e.g., Simply Cranberry brand)
		
		Beer, champagne, hard liquor (except rum), regular wine
		
		Diet sodas and soft drinks sweetened with approved sweeteners (see following list)
		
		Lemon juice and lime juice
		
		Lemonade sweetened with sugar
		
		Mexican or "Natural" sodas made with real sugar
		
		Milk (regular or lactose-free)
		
		Soft drinks or sports drinks sweetened with glucose or sugar
		
		Unsweetened nondairy milk substitutes:
		  Almond
		  Cashew
		  Coconut
		  Flax
		  Hemp
		  Oat
		  Pea protein–based
		  Rice
		
		Unsweetened tea and iced tea

Table 13-2 *(continued)*

	High-Fructose Foods (Avoid or Limit or Take Glucose Isomerase Enzyme Before Consuming)	Low-Fructose Foods (Enjoy as Desired)
Fruits and Veggies	Apples/applesauce	Apricot
	Asparagus	Banana
	Broccoli stalks (florets should be OK)	Berries
		Cantaloupe
	Cherries	Carambola (star fruit)
	Dried fruits, especially figs and mango (except for the small portions of dried fruits listed in the right column)	Citrus fruits (clementines, grapefruit, lemons, limes, oranges, tangerines)
		Dried fruit in 2 TBSP servings: dried cranberries, goji berries
	Figs	Grapes
	Mango	Guava
	Pear	Honeydew melon
	Watermelon	Kiwifruit
		Nectarine
		Papaya
		Passion fruit
		Peach
		Persimmon
		Pineapple
		Plum
		Pomegranate
		Tamarind

(continues)

Table 13-2 *(continued)*

	High-Fructose Foods (Avoid or Limit or Take Glucose Isomerase Enzyme Before Consuming)	Low-Fructose Foods (Enjoy as Desired)

Sweeteners and Ingredients	Agave nectar
	Allulose (?)*
	Corn syrup solids
	Fructose, crystalline fructose
	Fruit juice concentrates (e.g., apple, grape, pear)
	High-fructose corn syrup (HFCS)
	Honey
	Invert sugar
	Molasses
		100% maple syrup
		Brown rice syrup
		Brown sugar
		Corn syrup
		Dextrose
		Glucose
		Low-calorie sweeteners:
		  Acesulfame potassium
		  Aspartame
		  Monkfruit extract
		  Saccharin
		  Stevia
		  Sucralose (Splenda)
		White sugar (cane syrup, evaporated cane juice, sucrose, sugar)

Desserts and Sweets	Caramels Commercial baked goods made with HFCS Fruit chews/gummy candies Fruit compote Fruit leathers Fruit-filled danishes, pastries, and pies Honey-containing desserts, such as baklava Honey-containing granola/granola bars Honey-flavored cereals, cookies, etc. Lolliipops/natural/organic candies sweetened with fruit juice concentrates Sorbets or ice creams made with high-fructose fruits (mango, etc.)	Berry, coconut, or lemon ice creams and sorbets Commercial baked or homemade goods sweetened with sugar Premium ice cream sweetened with sugar

Table 13-2 *(continued)*

	High-Fructose Foods (Avoid or Limit or Take Glucose Isomerase Enzyme Before Consuming)	Low-Fructose Foods (Enjoy as Desired)
Condiments	BBQ sauces made with HFCS or honey Jams/jellies made with HFCS or honey Ketchup made with HFCS or honey Mango chutney Pancake syrup Relishes made with HFCS Salad dressings and marinades made with HFCS or honey Sweet Asian sauces: duck sauce, hoisin, plum sauce, sweet and sour sauce, teriyaki sauce Tomato sauce made with HFCS	100% lemon or lime juice 100% maple syrup Berry jams or orange marmalade made with real sugar Butter Herbs and spices Hot sauce (Tabasco, etc.) Mayonnaise Mustard Natural/organic ketchup made with sugar Oils Soy sauce Tomato sauce with no added sugar Vinegars

* **Allulose** is an increasingly popular low-calorie sweetener found in a variety of low-carb/keto packaged foods. It does not technically contain fructose, though it is chemically similar to fructose and is thought to be absorbed into the body by the same small intestinal transporters as fructose. Since people with fructose intolerance lack adequate transporters to absorb fructose, it is reasonable to worry that they would lack transporters to adequately absorb allulose, too. At the time of this writing, no studies have investigated allulose tolerance in fructose-intolerant people. Until more scientific data are available to clarify this issue, I've been advising my patients with fructose intolerance to avoid consuming allulose.

Low-Sucrose Diet

Best for:

- Sucrose intolerance or congenital sucrase-isomaltase deficiency (CSID)

- Temporary forms of sucrose intolerance caused by active celiac disease or Crohn's disease affecting the small intestine

Sucrose is a sugar that exists naturally in certain fruits, vegetables, and sweeteners like maple syrup and molasses. It can also be extracted from beets and sugar cane to derive isolated sugar that can be used as a sweetener. On a food label, it might also be listed as "cane juice" or "evaporated cane juice," but it's the same white stuff as plain old table sugar. Contrary to what you may have heard, brown-colored raw sugar or even brown sugar itself is not substantively different from white, more refined sugar—neither digestively nor metabolically. Sugar is sugar is sugar.

Sucrose intolerance is caused by inadequate production of the digestive enzyme called sucrase-isomaltase in your small intestine. Sucrase-isomaltase is required to break apart sucrose into its two component molecules, glucose and fructose, so they can be absorbed individually; see Figure 5-1 on page 83 for a visual of this process. When you consume more sucrose than you have the enzyme capacity to digest, the excess sucrose goes undigested and unabsorbed and travels to the colon, where it can cause gas, bloating, diarrhea, and cramping. Congenital sucrase-isomaltase deficiency (CSID) was once thought to be quite rare, especially so among adults, since CSID is a condition that is typically diagnosed in early childhood when a baby develops chronic diarrhea and fails to gain weight (failure to thrive). We now understand that there are many variants of sucrase-isomaltase-related genes, and certain ones that result in lower levels of enzyme production may be more prevalent among people who carry a diagnosis of IBS than among the general population. Relatedly, sucrose-intolerance can often be misdiagnosed as IBS.

CSID is considered a **primary sucrose intolerance**. However, some people temporarily lose the ability to digest sucrose when there has been damage to the enzyme-producing cells of the small intestine. This may happen in inflammatory conditions like uncontrolled celiac disease or active stages of Crohn's disease and is called **secondary sucrose intolerance**. Typically, secondary sucrose intolerance is reversed once healing of the affected segments of small intestine has taken place.

A low-sucrose diet is for people with sucrose intolerance who do not have access to supplemental enzymes that aid in sucrose digestion. On a low-sucrose diet, you can consume all animal proteins so long as they are not prepared with condiments, marinades, or other sugar-containing ingredients. Unsweetened dairy products are all also fine, so long as you're not also lactose intolerant. Nuts, seeds, butter, and vegetable oils are all fine. Some, but not all, people with sucrase-isomaltase deficiency can have a hard time digesting starchier foods as well, especially in larger portions. These include grains and starches like bread, pasta, flour-based baked goods, crackers, cereal, potatoes, rice, oatmeal, corn-based products, and chips/pretzels. If your symptoms are improved but not resolved on a low-sucrose diet, a one- to two-week elimination trial of grains and starches will tell you everything you need to know about whether these foods give you trouble as well. If the elimination trial resolves your symptoms, then gradual reintroduction with small amounts at a time will help you understand what portions you can consume comfortably. Chewing starchy foods for an extra-long time will help improve their absorbability by prolonging exposure to starch-digesting enzymes in the saliva.

Table 13-3: Low-Sucrose Diet for Sucrose Intolerance

	High-Sucrose Foods (Avoid or Limit or Take Prescription Sacrosidase Enzyme Before Consuming)	Low-Sucrose Foods (Enjoy as Desired)
Beverages and Liquids	All fruit juices (except unsweetened lemon/lime juice) Any sugar-sweetened beverages: flavored milks, iced tea, lemonade, sports drinks Fruit smoothies Regular sodas	Cappuccinos, regular milk (if not also lactose intolerant), or unsweetened lattes Coffee or tea (sweetened with approved sweeteners) Diet sodas or diet soft drinks Homemade iced tea/lemonade/ limeade sweetened with an approved sweetener (see following list)
Fruits	Apples Apricots Bananas Cantaloupe Dates Grapefruit Guava Honeydew Mango Nectarine Oranges (clementines, mandarins, tangelo, tangerines, etc.) Passion fruit Pineapple	Avocado Blackberries Blueberries Cherries Cranberries (fresh, not dried) Currants Figs (fresh, not dried) Grapes Kiwi Lemon Limes Pears Pomegranate Raspberries Rhubarb Strawberries

Table 13-3 *(continued)*

	High-Sucrose Foods (Avoid or Limit or Take Prescription Sacrosidase Enzyme Before Consuming)	Low-Sucrose Foods (Enjoy as Desired)
Vegetables and Legumes	Beans* (black, black eyed, kidney, lima, navy, pinto, etc.) Beets Butternut squash Carrots Cassava (yucca) Chickpeas/garbanzos Corn Edamame (boiled soybeans) Garlic Lentils Onions Parsnips Peas Potatoes Snow peas Split peas/dal Sweet potatoes Tempeh Tofu Yams	Alfalfa sprouts Artichoke Arugula Asparagus Bamboo shoots Bean sprouts (mung, soy) Bok choy Broccoli Brussels sprouts Cabbage Cauliflower Celery Chard Chives Collard greens Cucumber Eggplant Green beans/string beans Kale Lettuces (all) Mushrooms Okra Peppers Radish Spaghetti squash Spinach Tomatoes Turnips Yellow squash Zucchini

(continues)

Table 13-3 (continued)

	High-Sucrose Foods (Avoid or Limit or Take Prescription Sacrosidase Enzyme Before Consuming)	Low-Sucrose Foods (Enjoy as Desired)
Sweeteners and Ingredients	Sugar in all forms: 　Beet sugar 　Brown sugar 　Cane sugar 　Caramel 　Coconut sugar 　Confectioners' sugar 　Date sugar 　Maple syrup 　Molasses 　Raw sugar 　Sucanat 　Turbinado sugar	Agave nectar Dextrose (glucose) Fructose Low-calorie sweeteners: 　Acesulfame potassium 　Allulose 　Aspartame 　Monkfruit extract 　Saccharin 　Stevia 　Sucralose (Splenda) Sugar alcohols* or sweeteners that end with the letters _ol_ (erythritol, sorbitol, etc.) Pure/real honey (some varieties may be more tolerable than others) *These can cause digestive upset in some for reasons other than sucrose intolerance, however; see next section.

Table 13-3 *(continued)*

	High-Sucrose Foods (Avoid or Limit or Take Prescription Sacrosidase Enzyme Before Consuming)	Low-Sucrose Foods (Enjoy as Desired)
Desserts and Sweets	All baked goods, cakes, candies, chocolates, cookies, ice creams, pies, sorbets made with sugar or any of the sucrose-containing sweeteners previously listed	Homemade baked goods sweetened only with agave nectar or real honey Jell-O (Sugar Free) Keto or sugar-free chocolate bars (ChocZero) Sugar alcohol options for those who can tolerate: Fat Snax cookies and brownie bites HighKey keto cookies Jell-O (Sugar Free) pudding cups Rebel keto ice cream So Delicious no-sugar-added novelty pops (Dipped Vanilla Bean, Fudge Bars) SuperFat keto cookie bites

(continues)

Table 13-3 *(continued)*

	High-Sucrose Foods (Avoid or Limit or Take Prescription Sacrosidase Enzyme Before Consuming)	Low-Sucrose Foods (Enjoy as Desired)
Condiments	Almond/peanut butters with added sugar BBQ sauces made with sugar Chutneys Fruit preserves, jams, jellies, Ketchup Relishes Salad dressings and marinades made with sugar Sweet Asian sauces: duck sauce, hoisin, plum sauce, sweet and sour sauce, teriyaki sauce, etc. Tomato sauce made with garlic, onion, or sugar	100% lemon or lime juice Butter Herbs and spices Hot sauce (Tabasco, etc.) Mayonnaise Mustard Natural nut butters (no added sugar) Oils Soy sauce Vinegars

Low-Sugar Alcohol/Polyol Diets

Best for:

- People with chronic diarrhea of many origins that is not well controlled using fiber therapy or other interventions

- Including or especially IBS-D and inflammatory bowel disease (IBD)

Sugar alcohols, also known as polyols, are naturally occurring molecules that are similar in structure to sugar such that they taste sweet, but not similar enough to be absorbed into our bodies the same way that sugar is. This has a few implications. All human beings malabsorb sugar alcohols, and they will provoke diarrhea in anyone if a high-enough dose is consumed. Tolerance to sugar alcohols varies a lot by person; some people can consume a pretty substantial amount of them and feel fine, whereas more sensitive individuals can experience digestive upset—gas, bloating, and/or diarrhea—after consuming even tiny amounts.

Because sugar alcohols are not well absorbed, they barely affect blood sugar levels—if at all—and they contain fewer calories per gram than sugar. This makes sugar alcohols one of the more common sweeteners among keto products and other sugar-free/no-sugar-added products marketed to people with type 2 diabetes. Some packaged foods may list out the grams of sugar alcohols they contain as a separate line item on the "Nutrition Facts" label, but if not, you'll need to scan the ingredient list to alert you to their presence. Ingredients that end with the letters *ol* are sugar alcohols, and these include sorbitol, mannitol, maltitol, xylitol, erythritol, and lactitol. If you consume a large number of packaged, processed, low-carb/keto foods, your cumulative intake of sugar alcohols could get quite high, and this could provoke diarrhea on its own, though erythritol may be somewhat more tolerated than others of the sugar alcohols. In people experiencing diarrhea from another cause, even modest intakes of sugar alcohols can worsen their diarrhea. Celery juice is another dietary fad that can pile on sugar alcohols (mannitol) and aggravate diarrhea in susceptible people. I tend to steer my patients with chronic diarrhea away from sugar alcohols, though tolerance is often dose dependent, meaning that some people can often get away with eating small amounts of these foods.

Table 13-4: Low–Sugar Alcohol Diet for Chronic Diarrhea

	High in Sugar Alcohols (Avoid/Limit)	Low in Sugar Alcohols
Fruits and Juices	Apple cider or apple juice Apples (and applesauce) Apricot and pear juice/nectar Apricots Avocados Blackberries Celery juice Cherries Cranberry juice cocktail Diet or reduced calorie juices sweetened with sugar alcohols Dried fruits Green juices and smoothies made with apple or celery as a base Lychees Peaches Pears Plums Prune juice Tart cherry juice Watermelon	100% cranberry juice sweetened with sugar (Simply Cranberry brand) Bananas Blueberries Cantaloupe Citrus fruits (clementines, grapefruit, lemons, limes, oranges, tangerines) Figs Grapes Honeydew Kiwi Lemonade sweetened with sugar Mango Papaya Pineapple Raspberries Strawberries
Vegetables	Cauliflower Celery Mushrooms Sauerkraut Snow peas Sugar snap peas Sweet potatoes (larger portions)	All others not listed in left column

Table 13-4 *(continued)*

	High in Sugar Alcohols (Avoid/Limit)	Low in Sugar Alcohols
Sweeteners and Ingredients	Erythritol Erythritol-containing sweeteners, such as: Lakanto Swerve Truvia Isomal Lactitol Mannitol Maltitol Sorbitol Xylitol	All other sweeteners not listed in left column
Popular Low-Calorie, Low-Carb and Keto Treats and Condiments	Sugar-free condiments, such as: Jams and jellies Keto/low-carb protein bars No-sugar-added frozen yogurt; keto/sugar-free ice creams or sugar-free popsicles Pancake syrup Reduced calorie iced teas, juices, lemonades, and sodas Some brands of keto/low-carb breakfast cereal Sugar-free cakes and cookies Sugar-free candies, chocolates, and sugarless gum	Keto/low-carb products sweetened only with allulose, monkfruit, or stevia

(continues)

Table 13-4 *(continued)*

	High in Sugar Alcohols (Avoid/Limit)	Low in Sugar Alcohols
Medications and Supplements	Products commonly formulated with mannitol or sorbitol (check labels): Activated charcoal Beano (enzyme supplement) Chewable vitamins (especially kids' vitamins) Sublingual vitamin B$_{12}$	

Sugar-Restricted Diets for People with Multiple Carbohydrate Intolerances

If you have been diagnosed with multiple carbohydrate intolerances or are struggling with sensitivity to several sugars as the result of another condition, such as SIBO (Chapter 6), celiac disease (Chapter 6), or Crohn's disease (Chapter 7), then the fruits and vegetables most likely to be tolerated will have glucose as the predominant form of any sugar they do contain. The lists below highlight the fruits, vegetables, and sweeteners most likely to be tolerated by the absolute most sugar-sensitive of people.

Safest Fruits for People with Multiple Carbohydrate Intolerances (Low-Fructose, Low-Sucrose, and Low–Sugar Alcohols)

- Blueberries
- Grapes
- Kiwifruit
- Raspberries
- Strawberries

Safest Vegetables for People with Multiple Carbohydrate Intolerances (Low-Fructose, Low-Sucrose, and Low–Sugar Alcohols)

- Alfalfa sprouts
- Bok choy
- Broccoli (florets only, not stems)
- Chard
- Collard greens
- Cucumber
- Eggplant
- Green beans/string beans
- Kale
- Lettuces (all)
- Peppers
- Radishes
- Spaghetti squash
- Spinach
- Tomatoes (fresh, not tomato sauces or sun-dried tomatoes)
- Turnips
- Yellow/summer squash
- Zucchini

Safest Sweeteners for People with Multiple Carbohydrate Intolerances

(No Fructose, No Sucrose, and No Sugar Alcohols)

- Dextrose (granulated dextrose can be purchased and used instead of table sugar)
- Glucose syrup (often found as an ingredient in candies/confections)

- Karo Corn Syrup (this is 100% glucose)
- Monkfruit extract
- Stevia (Reb-A)
- Various artificial sweeteners: including aspartame and saccharin

Concluding Thoughts

GETTING REGULAR—AND STAYING REGULAR—MAY REQUIRE vastly different approaches for people experiencing problems with different causes (and frankly, even for two different people struggling with symptoms from the same cause!). As I've attempted to show you in this book, there are countless combinations of dietary interventions, dietary supplements, medications, and behavioral changes that may be helpful to you in your quest to conquer persistent diarrhea or constipation and gain control over your unruly bowels. Many of these interventions are things you can try on your own at home once you have an educated guess about what could be going on while others of them will require diagnostic and treatment assistance from a knowledgeable healthcare professional.

If you still feel unsure about what could be causing your issues after reading this book, and you have a pretty good sense that there's a direct link between your symptoms and specific food choices, it may be a good idea to maintain a detailed food and symptom diary for ten to fourteen days. While there are many apps that people use to track digestive symptoms vis-à-vis their diets, I will confess that most of them capture and present the data in ways that I find challenging to make much sense of. As a clinician, I really need to see the times of any symptoms my patients are experiencing in the context of the times they are eating various foods, and I need to see records for several days in a row to be able to make connections between, say, diarrhea in the morning to what might have been consumed the prior afternoon or evening. For me, this is easiest to visualize in the form of a very low-tech data table like the template below.

Sample Food and Symptom Journal Template

Date:			
Time	**Food and Beverage Consumed**	**Portion**	**Symptoms Experienced**
7:00 a.m.	Coffee + 2% milk + 1 orange	~½ cup milk in the coffee	
8:30 a.m.			Normal bowel movement
10:30 a.m.	1 whole wheat sandwich thin + cream cheese + 1 mini cucumber, sliced	~3 TBSP cream cheese	
12:30 p.m.	Ritter Sport brand milk chocolate with hazelnuts	4 squares	
2:30 p.m.	Roast beef sandwich with American cheese on a whole wheat sandwich thin		
4:00 p.m.			Normal bowel movement
7:00 p.m.	Chinese restaurant meal: chicken with broccoli, cold sesame noodles, white rice	Large portion of chicken/broccoli, ~½ cup noodles, ~1 cup rice	
7:30 p.m.			Lower-abdominal cramps, loose bowel movement
7:45 p.m.			Diarrhea

Medications/supplements taken today: gummy vitamin D 1,000 IU

When I am presented with specific, detailed data like the food journal example presented above, I can quickly start to develop hypotheses about what set off my patient's symptoms. In this sample case, there are a few possibilities that come to mind: Is he lactose intolerant, and could the undigested lactose from milk and milk chocolate he consumed early in the day be arriving in his colon immediately after dinner, propelled by ingesting his dinner meal (Chapter 5)? Or could this be an IBS-type situation where his higher-fat, larger dinner is overstimulating the digestive system's nerve reflexes, causing a bowel spasm (Chapter 4)? One day's worth of records won't answer the question, but with these two educated guesses, I can now comb the remaining week or two of food records I was provided to road test my hypothesis with other days and other meals to see if one of these ideas seems likelier than the other, or to see if a new idea emerges on reviewing other days.

In my experience, patients are pretty great at keeping detailed records for me, but they are typically less successful at drawing appropriate conclusions from the data they gather. A common mistake is to blame the food consumed immediately before a symptom appears as the cause of that symptom, when often symptoms may be caused by foods consumed one or two meals prior. When reactions follow specific meals quickly in a manner that does suggest a symptom was caused by something you just ate, people often blame the wrong food or ingredient. For example, diarrhea that kicks in immediately after ice cream gets blamed on lactose, not the impact of the fat. Diarrhea that kicks in immediately after an Italian pasta dinner usually gets blamed on the pasta (gluten; Chapter 6) rather than the tomato sauce (histamines; Chapter 8), garlic (FODMAPs; Chapters 4, 6), fat, or large portion (IBS triggers; Chapter 4) that accompanied it. In other cases, people are looking to pinpoint a specific food or ingredient intolerance to blame their symptoms on when the problem is more global—e.g., eating too much fiber in general when you struggle to empty your bowels adequately (Chapter 11). All this is to say that a well-seasoned GI-focused registered dietitian (or GI RD as we like to call ourselves) can help you make sense of the data you gather, and I encourage you to be open to exploring explanations for your symptoms that may not fit the narrative you've developed in your mind.

If your gastroenterologist doesn't have a great GI dietitian on their staff or on their speed dial (which they should!), you can consult the online database of expert GI dietitians hosted on the American Gastroenterological Association's website at https://patient .gastro.org. You can search for a dietitian by zip code, but now that telehealth is widely available, you may be able to work virtually with an expert dietitian from another state if you live in one of the twenty or so states that do not have exclusive practice laws for dietetics. Help is more accessible than ever, and no one with chronic bowel irregularity that affects their quality of life should have to "just live with it."

Glossary

^{13}C-sucrose breath test (SBT): A test used to diagnose sucrose intolerance that involves drinking a solution composed of sucrose that has been radiolabeled with a unique form of carbon called ^{13}C.

allulose: A low-calorie sweetener chemically similar to fructose. It cannot be metabolized for energy by the body's cells, which is why it has fewer calories than fructose and other sugars.

aminosalicylates (5-ASAs): Anti-inflammatory medications used to treat ulcerative colitis. Examples include mesalamine (Asacol, Pentasa, Lialda), sulfasalazine (Azulfidine), olsalazine (Dipentum), balsalazide (Colazal), and rectally administered medications like Rowasa or Canasa.

amylase: A starch-digesting enzyme produced by the pancreas.

anal fissure: A small tear in the skin and muscle lining your anus.

anaphylaxis: A severe, life-threatening allergic reaction that affects more than one system of the body at the same time.

anismus: Also known as dyssynergic defecation, anismus refers to abnormal coordination of the muscles that play a role in evacuating stool, resulting in an inability to evacuate stool effectively or completely.

anorectal manometry: A test used to diagnose pelvic floor dysfunction by measuring how well the anal sphincters coordinate to allow the effective passage of stool.

antibiotic: A medication that inhibits the growth of, or kills, microorganisms.

anticholinergic: A medication that slows down the colon's motility by inhibiting the action of acetylcholine, a chemical signaler between nerves and muscles.

antidiarrheal: A medication that reduces diarrhea. It may prevent excessive fluid and electrolyte secretions from the intestinal cells into the colon.

antihistamine: A medication that suppresses histamine's ability to affect the tissues of the body and prevent associated symptoms.

antispasmodic: A medication that interferes with nerve stimulation of involuntary (smooth) gut muscles.

atypical food allergy: An adverse food reaction carried out by the immune system, but that is not mediated by the same type of cells (IgE antibodies) responsible for typical food allergy reactions.

basophil: A type of white blood cell that is involved in many acute and chronic allergic reactions.

basophilia: A condition in which there is an excess of white blood cells called basophils in the bloodstream.

bile: A digestive fluid produced by the liver to aid in the digestion of fats and excretion of wastes.

bile acid: A component of the digestive fluid bile.

bile acid diarrhea (BAD): Diarrhea that results from bile acid malabsorption; also called cholerrhea.

bile acid malabsorption (BAM): A condition in which the body does not reabsorb bile acids, a component of digestive fluids, in the small intestine, resulting in excess amounts of them arriving to the colon and potentially causing bile acid diarrhea (BAD).

biofeedback therapy: A technique that is intended to help people gain conscious control over certain bodily functions. When used as a component of pelvic floor physical therapy, it can be helpful in treating dyssynergic defecation.

biologic: A medication composed of synthetic antibodies, usually given by intravenous or other injection methods, which actively target certain proteins that are fueling inflammation.

bowel: The intestines.

bowel movement: The act of passing stool (feces).

bowel regimen: A protocol of medications, supplements, behaviors, and/or routines collectively designed to promote a bowel movement.

brain-gut axis: The two-way communication channel that connects the central nervous system (brain) to the gastrointestinal tract.

breath testing: A noninvasive form of diagnostic testing that involves measuring hydrogen and methane gases in the breath following the ingestion of various substrates.

Bristol Stool Chart: A visual scale developed by Dr. Ken Heaton in the late 1990s that depicts various forms of stool, from type 1 to type 7, and that is used to aid the evaluation of constipation and diarrhea.

calprotectin: A protein found in the stool whose levels, when elevated, indicate intestinal inflammation.

carbohydrate intolerance: The diarrhea or other gastrointestinal symptoms that result from malabsorption of various sugars or sugar alcohols.

carbohydrate malabsorption: Incomplete absorption of a particular sugar in the small intestine, which results in undigested carbohydrate passing throughout the entirety of the bowel until defecation.

carcinoid tumor: A typically slow-growing, cancerous tumor that develops from neuroendocrine (hormone-producing) cells.

celiac disease: An autoimmune disease in which the body's immune cells launch a self-directed attack against the lining of the small intestine in response to ingestion of a protein called gluten, found in wheat, barley, rye, and other foods that may have come into contact with them.

chlorogenic acid: A natural chemical found in coffee that has a bowel-stimulating effect.

cholerrhea: Another name for bile acid diarrhea (see definition above).

chronic diarrhea: The persistence of loose stools for more than four weeks.

cognitive behavioral therapy (CBT): A solutions-oriented type of psychotherapy treatment that involves exploring how thoughts and emotions affect behaviors, and working to consciously change problematic thoughts that result in undesirable outcomes.

colectomy: A surgery that removes part or all of the colon (large intestine).

colitis: Any inflammation of the colon (large intestine).

colon: The large intestine, an approximately five-foot-long segment of the bowel that follows the small intestine, in which fluid, sodium, and potassium are reabsorbed into the body from the fecal stream. Undigested food matter (typically fiber) blends with other waste products to form stool in the large intestine, where it is stored until passage out of the body via the anus.

colonic inertia: A form of extremely slow colonic transit that results in severe constipation.

colonoscopy: A diagnostic procedure, typically conducted under sedation, in which a flexible endoscope is inserted into the large intestine via the anus so that the rectum, colon, and terminal ileum (tail end of the small intestine) can be visualized.

congenital sucrase-isomaltase deficiency (CSID): An inherited condition in which the body does not produce adequate levels of the enzyme sucrase-isomaltase, which is necessary to digest sugar (sucrose).

constipation: Difficulty emptying the bowels, characterized by infrequent stools (fewer than three per week), straining to defecate, and/or hard stools.

constipation-predominant irritable bowel syndrome (IBS-C): A disorder of the gut-brain interaction characterized by abdominal pain and hard, infrequent, and/or incomplete stools.

corticosteroid: Any hormone produced by the adrenal cortex or a synthetic hormone similar to the naturally occurring one. In gastrointestinal medicine, the term refers to an immune-system-suppressing medication chemically similar to cortisol that is used to treat various autoimmune conditions, including inflammatory bowel disease.

Crohn's disease: An autoinflammatory condition in which various segments of the gastrointestinal tract become inflamed, and often damaged, in ways that can affect nutrient absorption or the passage (motility) of food or waste.

CT scan: A type of computer-assisted X-ray imaging that shows cross sections of your insides, provides three-dimensional pictures, and offers more details, especially of soft tissues and blood vessels, than traditional X-ray imaging.

curcumin: An antioxidant-rich, bright yellow component of the culinary and medicinal herb turmeric that is sometimes used as a dietary supplement for its potential anti-inflammatory benefits.

dam-breaking diarrhea: A colloquial term coined at New York Gastroenterology Associates that describes diarrhea that follows multiple days of constipation or incomplete stool passage in which the diarrhea resembles a release of built-up pressure akin to that of a dam breaking.

dehydration: Inadequate fluid in the body to allow for proper physiologic function.

diamine oxidase (DAO): An enzyme that helps degrade a compound called histamine.

diaphragmatic breathing: Also known as belly breathing, a deep breathing technique used to help reduce the stress response.

diarrhea: The passage of loose or watery stools more than three times daily or in volumes of more than 200 g (~7 oz.) per day.

digestion: The process of breaking down food mechanically and chemically via enzymes within the gastrointestinal tract so the food's component parts can be absorbed and utilized by the body.

digestive enzyme: A protein that speeds up specific chemical reactions within the gastrointestinal tract to break apart large food molecules into smaller building blocks that can then be absorbed by the body.

digital rectal examination: An examination in which a healthcare provider inserts a gloved, lubricated finger into your rectum to feel for abnormalities.

disaccharidase: A digestive enzyme produced in the small intestine that has the capacity to break bonds between two-molecule sugars, such as lactose, sucrose, or maltose.

disaccharidase assay: A test that involves measuring the amount of disaccharidases (carbohydrate-digesting lactase, sucrase-isomaltase, maltase, and palatinase) in an intestinal biopsy sample. The sample is typically obtained by endoscopy.

disorder of the gut-brain interaction (DGBI): A condition that involves disturbances in the sensory or motor function of the gastrointestinal tract and how the brain processes stimuli that originate there.

diverticula: Small bulges in the inner lining of the intestinal wall that protrude outward through the muscle layer.

diverticulitis: Acute inflammation and infection of the diverticula.

diverticulosis: An asymptomatic condition in which there are diverticula present within the bowel.

dumping: Rapid emptying of the stomach's contents into the first segment of the small intestine that results in symptoms ranging from diarrhea and cramping to nausea, weakness, and fatigue.

dyssynergic defecation: Also known as anismus, this term refers to abnormal coordination of the muscles that play a role in evacuating stool, resulting in an inability to evacuate stool effectively or completely.

elastase: One of several protein-digesting enzymes produced by the pancreas whose abnormally low levels in the stool can be used to diagnose pancreatic insufficiency.

electrolyte: Minerals that carry an electric charge and play an essential role in maintaining fluid balance and cellular functions. Examples include sodium, potassium, chloride, calcium, and magnesium.

encopresis: A form of fecal incontinence in children that is related to constipation in which there is involuntary passage of stool into the underwear, also known as fecal soiling.

endoscopy: A diagnostic procedure conducted under sedation in which a flexible endoscope is inserted into the gastrointestinal tract. Upper endoscopy involves passing the endoscope into the mouth to visualize the esophagus, stomach, and/or early section of the small intestine (duodenum).

enema: Insertion of fluids into the rectum, typically as a remedy for constipation or for the administration of medications.

enteric-coated peppermint oil: Peppermint oil that is encapsulated in pills with specially designed coatings intended to resist breaking down in the stomach so that they arrive intact to the intestines to act locally there.

enzyme: A protein that facilitates specific chemical reactions without being changed by the reaction itself.

eosinophil: A white blood cell that plays a role in the immune system, particularly related to destroying parasitic infections and creating inflammation as part of the body's response to disease.

eosinophilic gastrointestinal disorders (EGIDs): A gastrointestinal disorder whose symptoms result from excessive numbers of eosinophils in the gastrointestinal tissue.

exclusive enteral nutrition (EEN): A liquid diet comprised solely of nutritionally complete beverages.

exocrine pancreatic insufficiency (EPI): A condition in which the pancreas does not release adequate levels of digestive enzymes and other secretions, such as bicarbonate. It may result in impaired digestion of carbohydrates, proteins, and/or fats.

fecal impaction: A hard mass of stool lodged in the colon or rectum that cannot pass through and that causes a blockage.

fecal incontinence: The involuntary passage of stool out of the anus, or the inability to hold in one's bowel movements.

fermentable: The susceptibility of a carbohydrate substance to being chemically broken down by bacteria or yeast.

fiber: A carbohydrate whose chemical bonds are unbreakable by human digestive enzymes, rendering it indigestible.

fiber supplement: A dietary supplement containing indigestible carbohydrates (fiber) used to provide a health benefit or improved functioning of the digestive tract.

fistula: An abnormal tunnel connecting the intestines and other adjacent structures, such as another piece of bowel, sometimes seen as a result of Crohn's disease.

food allergy: An adverse reaction to food carried out by the immune system as the result of mistaking a food protein for a harmful substance. Specifically, allergic reactions involve IgE antibodies triggering the release of histamine.

fructose intolerance: Adverse gastrointestinal symptoms, including diarrhea, cramping, gas or nausea, that result from poor absorption of the sugar fructose.

functional gastrointestinal disorder (FGID): A gastrointestinal disorder characterized by impaired sensory or motor function despite the absence of visible structural or objectively measurable causes for this dysfunction.

gastrocolic reflex (GCR): A digestive system reflex in which stretch of the stomach or arrival of fat into the small intestine activates motility in the colon.

gastrointestinal: Pertaining to the digestive tract, anywhere from the esophagus to the end of the intestines.

gentle fiber (GI gentle) diet: A soft-textured diet moderate in fiber that restricts raw vegetables and coarse, intact fiber from leafy vegetables, fruit/vegetable peels and skins, and whole nuts and seeds in favor of cooked, mechanically softer plant foods that are peeled, cooked, and/or pureed.

GI psychology: Also known as psychogastroenterology, an assortment of behavioral therapies intended to harness the brain as a partner in managing digestive symptoms and to provide people with behavioral and coping tools to improve health-related quality of life.

glucose isomerase: Also known as xylose isomerase, an enzyme that converts fructose to glucose.

L-glutamine: An amino acid or protein building block that is a preferred source of fuel for intestinal cells and supports their ability to multiply.

gluten: A protein found in wheat, barley, and rye, as well as other grains related to them.

glycerin suppository: An over-the-counter medication that takes the form of a small, waxy, bullet-shaped tablet inserted into the rectum for the purpose of stimulating a bowel movement or administering medication.

gut-directed hypnotherapy: A psychological therapy associated with GI psychology involving the induction of a deeply relaxed state whereby the brain is receptive to suggestions intended to produce changes in how it responds to gastrointestinal stimuli.

gut microbiota: The ecosystem of trillions of microorganisms that resides within the human gastrointestinal tract.

H$_1$ blocker: A type of antihistamine medication that works by preventing histamine from binding to certain types of receptors on the smooth muscle cells and tissues that line the blood vessels—all of which are involved in allergic-type reactions. When histamine attaches to such receptors, it can produce symptoms like itching, headaches, heart racing, swelling, reduced blood pressure (that can cause dizziness), difficulty breathing or airway constriction, and pain.

H$_2$ blocker: A type of antihistamine medication that works by preventing histamine from binding to certain types of receptors on the specialized stomach cells that produce stomach acid as well as to receptors throughout the small intestine. Using these medications can reduce acid production by the stomach and reduce symptoms of heartburn and chest pain related to acid reflux.

hemorrhoid: A cushion of tissue filled with veins within the anal canal.

histamine: A molecule released by white cells as part of an allergic or inflammatory response, causing blood vessels to become leaky and producing tissue swelling as a result.

histamine intolerance: An adverse reaction to consuming foods that are either high in preformed histamine, or that trigger the release of histamine, thought to be caused by an intestinal deficiency in a histamine-degrading enzyme called diamine oxidase (DAO).

hormone: A molecule produced at one location in the body and that travels via the bloodstream to serve as a chemical messenger for actions elsewhere in the body.

human milk oligosaccharide (HMO): Lab-made molecules that mimic prebiotics found in breast milk and that have been shown to foster the growth of beneficial species of bacteria (bifidobacteria) in the guts of infants.

hyperdefecation: Having frequent bowel movements, typically more than four times per day.

IBS-C: Constipation-predominant irritable bowel syndrome, a disorder of the gut-brain interaction characterized by abdominal pain associated with defecation and infrequent (fewer than three per week) bowel movements, straining to defecate, and/or hard stools.

immunomodulator: A medication that suppresses or otherwise alters the immune system, sometimes used to treat inflammatory bowel disease.

inflammatory bowel disease (IBD): Several autoinflammatory conditions in which various segments of the gastrointestinal tract become inflamed, and often damaged, in ways that can affect nutrient absorption or the passage (motility) of food or waste.

insoluble fiber: A form of dietary fiber that is not water soluble and that typically serves the role of adding bulk to stools due to its coarse texture.

inulin: A highly fermentable form of fiber. Inulin occurs naturally in some plant foods and may also be marketed as a prebiotic supplement or used as a food additive.

irregularity: The state of having inconsistent bowel patterns in terms of frequency of defecation and/or stool consistency.

irritable bowel syndrome (IBS-D): Diarrhea-predominant irritable bowel syndrome, a disorder of the gut-brain interaction characterized by abdominal pain associated with defecation and loose, urgent, and/or frequent bowel movements.

lactase enzyme: An enzyme produced in the small intestine that cleaves milk sugar (lactose) into its two component molecules, glucose and galactose, to render them absorbable.

lactose intolerance: Adverse gastrointestinal symptoms, including diarrhea, cramping, gas, or nausea, that result from poor absorption of milk sugar, or lactose.

lipase: A fat-digesting enzyme produced by the pancreas.

low-FODMAP diet: A therapeutic diet often used to manage symptoms of irritable bowel syndrome in which several categories of fermentable, poorly absorbed carbohydrates are avoided.

malabsorption: Impaired absorption of nutrients in the gastrointestinal tract.

malnutrition: Compromised health status as the result of inadequate intake or absorption of certain nutrients.

maltose intolerance: Adverse gastrointestinal symptoms, including diarrhea, cramping, gas, or nausea, that result from poor absorption of maltose, a sugar present in certain starchy foods.

mast cell disorder: A condition that causes abnormally high numbers of (or overactivity of) histamine-producing white blood cells called mast cells.

mast cell stabilizer: A medication used to treat mast cell disorders that inhibits histamine-producing white blood cells called mast cells from secreting too much histamine.

Mediterranean diet: A traditional dietary pattern characteristic of countries around the Mediterranean Sea that emphasizes fruits, vegetables, legumes, whole grains, and foods rich in unsaturated fats, such as nuts, olive oil, and fish.

metabolome: The sum total of metabolic by-products created by the gut microbiome.

motility: Movement or, when used in reference to the intestines, the rate of movement.

MR defecography: A test that utilizes MRI technology to visualize the pelvic floor muscles in action as they simulate defecation in order to evaluate their ability to coordinate. It is used to diagnose pelvic floor dysfunction.

neurotransmitter: A signaling molecule that functions as a chemical messenger between two nerves or between a nerve cell and another target cell.

obstruction: A blockage in the bowel that inhibits the passage of intestinal contents, gas, and/or stool.

osmotic diarrhea: A type of diarrhea that results from having a too-high concentration of unabsorbed substances in the colon that attract fluid from intestinal cells into the digestive tract through osmosis.

osmotic laxative: A laxative that works by drawing fluids into the colon via osmosis.

osmotic sugar: A sugar that has the potential to draw water across a semipermeable membrane through osmosis. In the digestive tract, this refers to unabsorbed sugars that arrive to the colon intact.

ostomy: A surgically created opening that connects the gastrointestinal tract to the outside of the body, such as the colon to the abdominal wall (colostomy).

outlet dysfunction: An umbrella term used to refer to any type of pelvic floor dysfunction that affects stool passage.

overflow diarrhea: Diarrhea that occurs in the setting of severe constipation in which fresher, liquid stool flows around an area of impacted or obstructive stool that cannot be dislodged.

partial enteral nutrition (PEN): A dietary regimen in which a portion of the day's calories are provided by nutritionally complete beverages instead of solid food.

pelvic floor: A group of muscles that support the pelvic organs (uterus, vagina, cervix, bladder, urethra, and rectum) and play a role in defecation, urination, and sexual function.

pelvic floor dysfunction: Abnormal function of one or more of the pelvic floor muscles that affects defecation, urination, and/or sexual function.

pelvic floor dyssynergia: A particular type of pelvic floor dysfunction in which faulty coordination of the anal sphincter muscles results in defecation problems.

pelvic floor physical therapy: A specialty form of physical therapy that focuses on rehabilitation and/or retraining of the pelvic floor muscles to treat pelvic floor dysfunction.

polyols: Also known as sugar alcohols, a family of sweet-tasting carbohydrates that are poorly absorbed in the human digestive tract and therefore do not contribute a substantial amount of calories to the diet.

postbiotic: A term that refers to short-chain fatty acids (compounds produced by microorganisms in the gut microbiota) or inactivated microorganisms themselves, which have been demonstrated to confer a health benefit when ingested.

post-infectious IBS (IBS-PI): A form of irritable bowel syndrome whose onset is in the immediate aftermath of an acute gastrointestinal infection.

pouchitis: Inflammation of the surgically created intestinal pouch following a total proctocolectomy for ulcerative colitis.

prebiotic: A type of fiber that is fermentable by members of the *Lactobacillus* and *Bifidobacterium* genera and, when consumed, promotes their growth within the gut microbiota.

primary lactose intolerance: Lactose intolerance that results from genetically programmed reductions in lactase enzyme production among the cells lining the small intestine.

primary sucrose intolerance: Sucrose intolerance that results from genetically programmed reductions in sucrase-isomaltase enzyme production among the cells lining the small intestine.

probiotic: Live microorganisms that have been documented to confer a health benefit on their host.

protease: A protein-digesting enzyme, often produced by the pancreas.

protein: An organic (carbon-containing) molecule composed of amino acids as building blocks. Proteins form many of the essential structures, enzymes, and immune mediators necessary for life. Nutritionally, protein is one of the three major macronutrients (energy-providing nutrients) in the human diet and is the only one that contains nitrogen.

pylorus: The passageway between the stomach and the first segment of the small intestine (duodenum).

rectal suppository: A small, bullet-shaped medication administered via the rectum to help stimulate defecation.

rectocele: A weakness in the muscular back wall of the vagina that separates it from the rectum. When a person strains to defecate or urinate, the weakness may bulge from the rectum into the vagina. The bulge creates a pocket where stool can get lodged on its way out, making it difficult to completely empty.

rectum: The final, straight segment of the large intestine (colon).

regularity: Refers to bowel regularity, and describes the situation in which a person experiences predictable patterns of satisfactory bowel movements.

remission: A temporary cessation or quieting of disease activity in the setting of a chronic disease.

Rome Criteria: Consensus-based criteria developed by the Rome Foundation (North Carolina, USA) to diagnose functional gastrointestinal disorders.

secondary lactose intolerance: A temporary and reversible form of lactose intolerance that results from damage to the lactase-producing cells lining the small intestine.

secondary sucrose intolerance: A temporary and reversible form of lactose intolerance that results from damage to the sucrase-isomaltase-producing cells lining the small intestine.

secretagogue: A medication used to treat constipation that acts by increasing secretion of electrolytes and water by the cells that line the colon. This softens stools and increases movement within the bowel.

serotonergic agent: A medication that affects bowel motility by altering peristalsis—or waves of muscular contractions—by activating one or more serotonin receptors in the gut and its nerves.

serotonin: A neurotransmitter produced by cells lining the intestine that plays a key role in communicating information to the brain about what is occurring in the gut.

Sitz bath: A shallow basin that can attach to a toilet seat allowing the buttocks to be immersed in warm water for the purpose of relieving pain associated with anal fissures or symptomatic hemorrhoids.

Sitz marker test: A motility test used to measure transit time through the colon and diagnose slow transit constipation. It entails swallowing a capsule that contains tiny markers that can be tracked via X-rays as they make their way through the colon.

slow transit constipation: Constipation caused by abnormally prolonged transit time.

small intestinal bacterial overgrowth (SIBO): The presence of an abnormally high concentration of bacteria (more than 1,000 colony-forming units of bacteria per milliliter of secretions) in the early part of the jejunum, a region of the small intestine.

SmartPill: A method of evaluating whole-gut motility that involves swallowing a single-use pill that contains sensors that wirelessly transmit data to a receiver worn outside the body.

soluble fiber: A form of dietary fiber that dissolves in water, improving the water-holding properties of stool and slowing down excessively rapid colonic transit time as a result of its viscosity.

soluble fiber therapy: The therapeutic use of soluble fiber–rich foods and/or supplements to promote more formed, regular bowel movements; it is typically used to manage looser stools and diarrhea.

specific carbohydrate diet (SCD): A grain-free, low-sugar, low-dairy diet that was popularized in the 1990s in a book called *Breaking the Vicious Cycle* and that is sometimes used to help manage symptoms of inflammatory bowel disease.

steatorrhea: A type of diarrhea resulting from unabsorbed fat.

stimulant laxative: A medication used to treat constipation that works by causing the colon to contract more regularly and/or strongly.

stool: The fecal material that makes up a bowel movement.

stool burden: The amount of retained stool in the colon. This is increased by chronically incomplete stool passage/constipation.

stool softener: A medication used to soften stools that works by lowering the surface tension of stool, which allows more water to enter into it.

stricture: A narrowing of the tubular intestinal tract that may occur as a direct result of inflammation, and that can cause blockages when certain textures of fiber are consumed.

sucrose: A type of sugar found naturally in sugarcane, beets, maple syrup, certain vegetables (carrots, corn, onions, garlic, potatoes) and many fruits. Chemically, it is composed of a glucose and a fructose molecule joined together.

sucrose intolerance: Adverse gastrointestinal symptoms, including diarrhea, cramping, gas, and nausea, that result from poor absorption of the sugar sucrose.

sugar alcohol: Also known as a polyol, a family of sweet-tasting carbohydrates that are poorly absorbed in the human digestive tract and therefore do not contribute a substantial amount of calories to the diet.

terminal ileum: The tail end of the small intestine, immediately proximal to the colon. It is about thirty centimeters long.

toileting position: The physical position one assumes when sitting on a toilet.

total proctocolectomy: A surgery in which the entire colon and rectum are removed.

transenteric scintigraphy: A method of evaluating whole-gut motility that involves swallowing a radiolabeled meal whose journey can be tracked and timed using a special camera.

tricyclic antidepressant (TCA): A class of antidepressant medication that is used "off-label" at low doses to manage gastrointestinal pain and irregular bowel function.

ulcerative colitis: An autoinflammatory condition in which the rectum and colon become inflamed, and often damaged, in ways that can affect the passage (motility) of waste and reabsorption of fluids and electrolytes.

vaginal splinting: The insertion of a finger or fingers into the vagina to press against the back wall in order to facilitate the completion of a bowel movement. This technique can be helpful for people with rectoceles who experience difficulty eliminating complete bowel movements.

vaginal suppository: A small, bullet-shaped medication inserted into the vagina.

visceral hypersensitivity: Having a lower-than-average threshold for pain or discomfort related to stimuli within the gastrointestinal tract.

xylose isomerase: Also known as glucose isomerase, an enzyme that converts fructose to glucose.

References

LISTED BELOW ARE THE PRINCIPAL sources that I consulted in preparing this book and upon which much of my clinical approach is based.

In addition to the sources listed below, I referenced the product labels and/or company websites of foods and name-brand medicines and dietary supplements referenced throughout this manuscript for information on dosing as well as active and inactive ingredients. The information cited was current as of December 2021.

Chapter 1

Lewis SJ, Heaton KW. Stool form scale as a useful guide to intestinal transit time. *Scand J Gastroenterol*. 1997;32(9):920–924.

Rose C, Parker A, Jefferson B, Cartmell E. The characterization of feces and urine: A review of the literature to inform advanced treatment technology. *Crit Rev Environ Sci Technol*. 2015;45(17):1827–1879.

Chapter 2

Hofmann AF. The continuing importance of bile acids in liver and intestinal disease. *Arch Intern Med*. 1999;159(22):2647–2658.

Mailhe M, Ricaboni D, Vitton V, et al. Repertoire of the gut microbiota from stomach to colon using culturomics and next-generation sequencing. *BMC Microbiol*. 2018;18:157.

Seeley R, Stephens T, Tate P. *Essentials of Anatomy & Physiology* (6th ed.). New York: McGraw Hill; 2006.

Chapter 4

Altobelli E, Del Negro V, Angeletti PM, Latella G. Low-FODMAP diet improves irritable bowel syndrome symptoms: A meta-analysis. *Nutrients.* 2017 Aug;9(9):940.

Camilleri M. Serotonergic modulation of visceral sensation: Lower gut. *Gut.* 2002;51:i81–i86.

Dale HF, Rasmussen SH, Asiller ÖÖ, Lied GA. Probiotics in irritable bowel syndrome: An up-to-date systematic review. *Nutrients.* 2019 Sep;11(9):2048.

Fritscher-Ravens A, Pflaum T, Mösinger M, et al. Many patients with irritable bowel syndrome have atypical food allergies not associated with immunoglobulin E. *Gastroenterology.* 2019;157(1):109–118.e5.

Gibson P, Shepherd S. Evidence-based dietary management of functional gastrointestinal symptoms: The FODMAP approach. *J Gastroenterol Hepatol.* 2010;25(2):252–258.

Gibson P. The evidence base for efficacy of the low FODMAP diet in irritable bowel syndrome: Is it ready for prime time as a first-line therapy? *J Gastroenterol Hepatol.* 2017;32 Suppl (1):32–35.

Gleeson M. Dosing and efficacy of glutamine supplementation in human exercise and sport training. *J Nutr.* 2008;138(10):2045S-2049S.

Gunn D, Abbas Z, Harris HC, Major G, Hoad C, Gowland P, Marciani L, Gill SK, Warren FJ, Rossi M, Remes-Troche JM, Whelan K, Spiller RC. Psyllium reduces inulin-induced colonic gas production in IBS: MRI and *in vitro* fermentation studies. *Gut.* 2021 Aug 5:gutjnl-2021-324784.

Holscher HD, Doligale JL, Bauer LL, Gourineni V, Pelkman CL, Fahey GC, Swanson KS. Gastrointestinal tolerance and utilization of agave inulin by healthy adults. *Food Funct.* 2014 Jun;5(6):1142–1149.

Kato O, Misawa H. Treatment of diarrhea-predominant irritable bowel syndrome with paroxetine. *Prim Care Companion J Clin Psychiatry.* 2005;7(4):202.

Keefer L, Palsson OS, Pandolfino JE. Best practice update: Incorporating psychogastroenterology into management of digestive disorders. *Gastroenterology.* 2018 Apr;154(5):1249–1257.

Khanna R, MacDonald JK, Levesque BG. Peppermint oil for the treatment of irritable bowel syndrome: A systematic review and meta-analysis. *J Clin Gastroenterol.* 2014 Jul;48(6):505–512.

Klem F, Wadhwa A, Prokop LJ, et al. Prevalence, risk factors, and outcomes of irritable bowel syndrome after infectious enteritis: A systematic review and meta-analysis. *Gastroenterology.* 2017;152(5):1042–1054.e1.

Lembo A, Pimentel M, Rao SS, et al. Repeat treatment with rifaximin is safe and effective in patients with diarrhea-predominant irritable bowel syndrome. *Gastroenterology.* 2016; 151(6):1113–1121.

O'Mahony L, McCarthy J, Kelly P, Hurley G, Luo F, Chen K, O'Sullivan GC, Kiely B, Collins JK, Shanahan F, Quigley EM. *Lactobacillus* and *Bifidobacterium* in irritable bowel syndrome: Symptom responses and relationship to cytokine profiles. *Gastroenterology.* 2005;128(3):541–551.

Ormsbee HS 3rd, Fondacaro JD. Action of serotonin on the gastrointestinal tract. *Proc Soc Exp Biol Med.* 1985 Mar;178(3):333–338.

Palsson OS, Peery A, Seitzberg D, Amundsen ID, McConnell B, Simrén M. Human milk oligosaccharides support normal bowel function and improve symptoms of irritable bowel syndrome: A multicenter, open-label trial. *Clin Transl Gastroenterol.* 2020 Dec;11(12):e00276.

Palsson OS, Whitehead WE. Hormones and IBS. University of North Carolina Center for Functional and GI Motility Disorders website. https://www.med.unc.edu/ibs/wp-content/uploads/sites/450/2017/10/IBS-and-Hormones.pdf. Accessed December 12, 2021.

Pimentel M, Lembo A, Chey WD, et al. Rifaximin therapy for patients with irritable bowel syndrome without constipation. *N Engl J Med.* 2011;364(1):22–32.

Schmick M, Hornecker J. Irritable bowel syndrome: A review of treatment options. *US Pharm.* 2017;42(12):20–26.

Su GL, Ko CW, Bercik P, et al. AGA Clinical practice guidelines on the role of probiotics in the management of gastrointestinal disorders. *Gastroenterology.* 2020;159(2):697–705.

Surdea-Blaga T, Baban A, Nedelcu L, Dumitrascu DL. Psychological interventions for irritable bowel syndrome. *J Gastrointestin Liver Dis.* 2016 Sep;25(3):359–366.

Vulevic J, Tzortzis G, Juric A, Gibson GR. Effect of a prebiotic galactooligosaccharide mixture (B-GOS®) on gastrointestinal symptoms in adults selected from a general population who suffer with bloating, abdominal pain, or flatulence. *Neurogastroenterol Motil.* 2018 Nov;30(11):e13440.

Vulevic J, Drakoularakou A, Yaqoob P, Tzortzis G, Gibson GR. Modulation of the fecal microflora profile and immune function by a novel trans-galactooligosaccharide mixture (B-GOS) in healthy elderly volunteers. *Am J Clin Nutr.* 2008 Nov;88(5):1438–1446.

Whorwell PJ, Altringer L, Morel J, Bond Y, Charbonneau D, O'Mahony L, Kiely B, Shanahan F, Quigley EM. Efficacy of an encapsulated probiotic *Bifidobacterium infantis* 35624 in women with irritable bowel syndrome. *Am J Gastroenterol*. 2006;101(7):1581–1590.

Wilson B, Whelan K. Prebiotic inulin-type fructans and galacto-oligosaccharides: Definition, specificity, function, and application in gastrointestinal disorders. *J Gastroenterol Hepatol*. 2017 Mar;32 Suppl 1:64–68.

Zhou Q, Verne ML, Fields JZ, et al. Randomised placebo-controlled trial of dietary glutamine supplements for postinfectious irritable bowel syndrome. *Gut*. 2019; 68:996–1002.

Chapter 5

Gao KP, Mitsui T, Fujiki K, Ishiguro H, Kondo T. Effects of lactase preparations in asymptomatic individuals with lactase deficiency—gastric digestion of lactose and breath hydrogen analysis. *J Med Sci*. 2002;65(1–2):21–28.

Garcia-Etxebarria K, Zheng T, Bonfiglio F, et al. Increased prevalence of rare sucrase-isomaltase pathogenic variants in irritable bowel syndrome patients. *Clin Gastroenterol Hepatol*. 2018;16(10):1673–1676.

Gibson PR, Newnham E, Barrett JS, Shepherd SJ, Muir JG. Review article: Fructose malabsorption and the bigger picture. *Aliment Pharmacol Ther*. 2007;25(4):349–363.

Kim SB, Calmet FH, Garrido J, Garcia-Buitrago MT, Moshiree B. Sucrase-isomaltase deficiency as a potential masquerader in irritable bowel syndrome. *Dig Dis Sci*. 2020;65(2):534–540.

Komericki P, Akkilic-Materna M, Strimitzer T, Weyermair K, Hammer HF, Aberer W. Oral xylose isomerase decreases breath hydrogen excretion and improves gastrointestinal symptoms in fructose malabsorption—a double-blind, placebo-controlled study. *Aliment Pharmacol Ther*. 2012;36(10):980–987.

Levine B, Weisman S. Enzyme replacement as an effective treatment for the common symptoms of complex carbohydrate intolerance. *Nutr Clin Care*. 2004;7(2):75–81.

Lin MY, Dipalma JA, Martini MC, Gross CJ, Harlander SK, Savaiano DA. Comparative effects of exogenous lactase (beta-galactosidase) in preparations on in vivo lactose digestion. *Dig Dis Sci*. 1993; 38(11):2022–2027.

Robayo-Torres CC, Opekun AR, Quezada-Calvillo R, et al. 13C-breath tests for sucrose digestion in congenital sucrase isomaltase-deficient and sacrosidase-supplemented patients. *J Pediatr Gastroenterol Nutr*. 2009;48(4):412–418.

Sanders SW, Tolmac KG, Reitberg DP. Effect of a single dose of lactase on symptoms and expired hydrogen after lactose challenge in lactose-intolerant subjects. *Clin Pharm.* 1992;11(6):533–538.

Chapter 6

Apte MV, Wilson JS, Korsten MA. Alcohol-related pancreatic damage: Mechanisms and treatment. *Alcohol Health Res World.* 1997;21(1):13–20.

Bures J, Cyrany J, Kohoutova D, et al. Small intestinal bacterial overgrowth syndrome. *World J Gastroenterol.* 2010;16(24):2978–2990.

Camilleri M, Vijayvargiya P. The role of bile acids in chronic diarrhea. *Am J Gastroenterol.* 2020;115(10):1596–1603.

Camilleri M. Bile acid diarrhea: Prevalence, pathogenesis, and therapy. *Gut Liver.* 2015;9(3):332–339. doi:10.5009/gnl14397.

Chedid V, Dhalla S, Clarke JO, et al. Herbal therapy is equivalent to rifax-imin for the treatment of small intestinal bacterial overgrowth. *Glob Adv Health Med.* 2014;3(3):16–24.

Choung RS, Ditah IC, Nadeau AM, et al. Trends and racial/ethnic dispar-ities in gluten-sensitive problems in the United States: Findings from the National Health and Nutrition Examination surveys from 1988 to 2012. *Am J Gastroenterol.* 2015;110(3):455–461.

Gottlieb K, Wacher V, Sliman J, Pimentel M. Review article: Inhibition of methanogenic archaea by statins as a targeted management strat-egy for constipation and related disorders. *Aliment Pharmacol Ther.* 2016;43(2):197–212.

Häuser W, Musial F, Caspary WF, Stein J, Stallmach A. Predictors of irri-table bowel-type symptoms and healthcare-seeking behavior among adults with celiac disease. *Psychosom Med.* 2007;69(4):370–376.

Krigel A, Turner KO, Makharia GK, Green PH, Genta RM, Leb-wohl B. Ethnic variations in duodenal villous atrophy consistent with celiac disease in the United States. *Clin Gastroenterol Hepatol.* 2016;14(8):1105–1111.

Leite GGS, Weitsman S, Parodi G, et al. Mapping the segmental mi-crobiomes in the human small bowel in comparison with stool: A REIMAGINE study. *Dig Dis Sci.* 2020;65(9):2595–2604.

Meijer C, Shamir R, Szajewska H, Mearin L. Celiac disease prevention. *Front Pediatr.* 2018;6:368.

Monash University FODMAP Diet app. Version 3.0.8 (434). Monash University.

Muskal SM, Sliman J, Kokai-Kun J, Pimentel M, Wacher V, Gottlieb K. Lovastatin lactone may improve irritable bowel syndrome with constipation (IBS-C) by inhibiting enzymes in the archaeal methano-genesis pathway. *F1000Res.* 2016 Apr;5:606.

Pimentel M, Saad RJ, Long MD, Rao SSC. ACG Clinical guide-line: Small intestinal bacterial overgrowth. *Am J Gastroenterol.* 2020;115(2):165–178.

Rezaie A, Buresi M, Lembo A, et al. Hydrogen and methane-based breath testing in gastrointestinal disorders: The North American consensus. *Am J Gastroenterol.* 2017;112(5):775–784.

Shah SC, Day LW, Somsouk M, Sewell JL. Meta-analysis: Antibiotic ther-apy for small intestinal bacterial overgrowth. *Aliment Pharmacol Ther.* 2013;38(8):925–934.

Smolka AJ, Schubert ML. *Helicobacter pylori*–induced changes in gastric acid secretion and upper gastrointestinal disease. *Curr Top Microbiol Immunol.* 2017;400:227–252.

Synthetic Biologics Inc. Synthetic biologics provides update on investigator-sponsored phase 2b clinical study of SYN-010 in IBS-C patients. Available at www.prnewswire.com/news-releases/synthetic-biologics -provides-update-on-investigator-sponsored-phase-2b-clinical-study -of-syn-010-in-ibs-c-patients-301144645.html. Accessed January 2, 2022.

Vici G, Camilletti D, Polzonetti V. Possible role of vitamin D in celiac dis-ease onset. *Nutrients.* 2020 Apr;12(4):1051. doi:10.3390/nu12041051.

Vijayvargiya P, Camilleri M. Update on bile acid malabsorption: Ready for prime time? *Curr Gastroenterol Rep.* 2018;20(3):10.

Vijayvargiya P, Gonzalez Izundegui D, Calderon G, Tawfic S, Batbold S, Camilleri M. Fecal bile acid testing in assessing patients with chronic unexplained diarrhea: Implications for healthcare utilization. *Am J Gastroenterol.* 2020;115(7):1094–1102.

Chapter 7

Chandan S, Mohan BP, Chandan OC, et al. Curcumin use in ulcerative colitis: Is it ready for prime time? A systematic review and meta-analysis of clinical trials. *Ann Gastroenterol.* 2020;33(1):53–58.

Dang X, Xu M, Liu D, Zhou D, Yang W. Assessing the efficacy and safety of fecal microbiota transplantation and probiotic VSL#3 for active ulcerative colitis: A systematic review and meta-analysis. *PLoS One.* 2020;15(3):e0228846.

Griffin N, Grant LA, Anderson S, Irving P, Sanderson J. Small bowel MR enterography: Problem solving in Crohn's disease. *Insights Imaging.* 2012;3(3):251–263.

Heerasing N, Thompson B, Hendy P, et al. Exclusive enteral nutrition provides an effective bridge to safer interval elective surgery for adults with Crohn's disease. *Aliment Pharmacol Ther*. 2017;45(5):660–669.

Levine A, Rhodes JM, Lindsay JO, et al. Dietary guidance from the International Organization for the Study of Inflammatory Bowel Diseases. *Clin Gastroenterol Hepatol*. 2020;18(6):1381–1392.

Lewis JD, Sandler RS, Brotherton C, et al. A randomized trial comparing the specific carbohydrate diet to a Mediterranean diet in adults with Crohn's disease. *Gastroenterology*. 2021;161(3):837–852.e9.

Manitius N. Fiber for Inflammatory Bowel Disease (patient education handout). Dietitians in Medical Nutrition Therapy, a dietetic practice group of the Academy of Nutrition and Dietetics. 2021.

Narula N, Wong ECL, Dehghan M, et al. Association of ultra-processed food intake with risk of inflammatory bowel disease: Prospective cohort study. *BMJ*. 2021;374:n1554.

Nguyen DL, Palmer LB, Nguyen ET, McClave SA, Martindale RG, Bechtold ML. Specialized enteral nutrition therapy in Crohn's disease patients on maintenance infliximab therapy: A meta-analysis. *Therap Adv Gastroenterol*. 2015;8(4):168–175.

Su GL, Ko CW, Bercik P, et al. AGA clinical practice guidelines on the role of probiotics in the management of gastrointestinal disorders. *Gastroenterology*. 2020;159(2):697–705.

Chapter 8

Chin KW, Garriga MM, Metcalfe DD. The histamine content of oriental foods. *Food Chem Toxicol*. 1989;27(5):283–287.

Chung BY, Cho SI, Ahn IS, et al. Treatment of atopic dermatitis with a low-histamine diet. *Ann Dermatol*. 2011;23 Suppl 1:S91–S95.

Comas-Basté O, Sánchez-Pérez S, Veciana-Nogués MT, Latorre-Moratalla M, Vidal-Carou MDC. Histamine intolerance: The current state of the art. *Biomolecules*. 2020;10(8):1181.

Feldman JM. Histaminuria from histamine-rich foods. *Arch Intern Med*. 1983;143(11):2099–2102.

Ganesh A, Maxwell LG. Pathophysiology and management of opioid-induced pruritus. *Drugs*. 2007;67(16):2323–2333.

Hermens JM, Hanifin JM, Hirschman CA. Comparison of histamine release in human skin mast cells induced by morphine and fentanyl as supplements to nitrous oxide anesthesia. *Anesthesiology*. 1985;62:124–129.

Hrubisko M, Danis R, Huorka M, Wawruch M. Histamine intolerance—the more we know the less we know. A review. *Nutrients*. 2021;13(7):2228.

Joneja JV. *Dealing with Food Allergies: A Practical Guide to Detecting Culprit Foods and Eating a Healthy, Enjoyable Diet.* Bull Publishing Company; 2003.

Joneja JV. *Histamine Intolerance: A Comprehensive Guide for Healthcare Professionals.* 1st ed. Lawrence H, ed. Berrydale Books; 2017.

Komericki P, et al. Histamine intolerance: Lack of reproducibility of single symptoms by oral provocation with histamine: A randomised, double-blind, placebo-controlled cross-over study. *Wiener Klinische Wochenschrift.* 2011; 123(1–2):15–20.

Leitner R, Zoernpfenning E, Missbichler A. Evaluation of the inhibitory effect of various drugs/active ingredients on the activity of human diamine oxidase *in vitro. Clin Transl Allergy.* 2014;4(Suppl 3):P23.

Maintz L, et al. Evidence for a reduced histamine degradation capacity in a subgroup of patients with atopic eczema. *J Allergy Clin Immunol.* 2006;117.5:1106–1112.

Manzotti G, Breda D, Di Gioacchino M, Burastero SE. Serum diamine oxidase activity in patients with histamine intolerance. *Int J Immunopath Pharmacol.* 2016;29:105–111.

McNicol E, Horowicz-Mehler N, Fisk RA. Management of opioid side effects in cancer-related and chronic noncancer pain: A systematic review. *Journal of Pain.* 2003;4(5):231–256.

Reese I, Ballmer-Weber B, Beyer K, et al. German guideline for the management of adverse reactions to ingested histamine: Guideline of the German Society for Allergology and Clinical Immunology (DGAKI), the German Society for Pediatric Allergology and Environmental Medicine (GPA), the German Association of Allergologists (AeDA), and the Swiss Society for Allergology and Immunology (SGAI). *Allergo J Int.* 2017;26(2):72–79.

Sánchez-Pérez S, Comas-Basté O, Rabell-González J, Veciana-Nogués MT, Latorre-Moratalla ML, Vidal-Carou MC. Biogenic amines in plant-origin foods: Are they frequently underestimated in low-histamine diets? *Foods.* 2018;7(12):205.

Schink M, Konturek PC, Tietz E, et al. Microbial patterns in patients with histamine intolerance. *J Physiol Pharmacol.* 2018;69(4):10.26402/jpp.2018.4.09.

Schnedl WJ, Enko D. Histamine intolerance originates in the gut. *Nutrients.* 2021;13(4):1262.

Schnedl WJ, Schenk M, Lackner S, Enko D, Mangge H, Forster F. Diamine oxidase supplementation improves symptoms in patients with histamine intolerance. *Food Sci. Biotechnol.* 2019;28:1779–1784.

Schwelberger, HG. Histamine intolerance: A metabolic disease? *Inflamm Res.* 2010; 59.2:219–221.

Slorach SA. Chapter 15, Histamine in Food. In: Uvnäs B, ed. *Histamine and Histamine Agonists.* Springer-Verlag Berlin Heidelberg; 1991.

Son JH, Chung BY, Kim HO, Park CW. A histamine-free diet is helpful for treatment of adult patients with chronic spontaneous urticaria. *Ann Dermatol.* 2018;30(2):164–172.

Tuck CJ, Biesiekierski JR, Schmid-Grendelmeier P, Pohl D. Food intolerances. *Nutrients.* 2019;11(7):1684.

University of Maryland Medical Center Website. Quercetin. http://accurateclinic.com/wp-content/uploads/2016/02/Quercetin-University-of-Maryland-Medical-Center.pdf. Accessed December 12, 2021.

Wantke F, Götz M, Jarisch R. The red wine provocation test: Intolerance to histamine as a model for food intolerance. *Allergy and Asthma Proceedings.* 1994;15(1).

Wöhrl, S, et al. Histamine intolerance-like symptoms in healthy volunteers after oral provocation with liquid histamine. *Allergy and Asthma Proceedings.* 2004;25(5).

Chapter 9

Grooms KN, Ommerborn MJ, Pham DQ, Djoussé L, Clark CR. Dietary fiber intake and cardiometabolic risks among US adults, NHANES 1999–2010. *Am J Med.* 2013;126(12):1059–67.e674.

Kranz S, Brauchla M, Slavin JL, Miller KB. What do we know about dietary fiber intake in children and health? The effects of fiber intake on constipation, obesity, and diabetes in children. *Adv Nutr.* 2012;3(1):47–53.

Lambeau KV, McRorie JW Jr. Fiber supplements and clinically proven health benefits: How to recognize and recommend an effective fiber therapy. *J Am Assoc Nurse Pract.* 2017;29(4):216–223.

Chapter 10

Bayer SB, Gearry RB, Drummond LN. Putative mechanisms of kiwifruit on maintenance of normal gastrointestinal function. *Crit Rev Food Sci Nutr.* 2018;58(14):2432–2452.

Chang CC, Lin YT, Lu YT, Liu YS, Liu JF. Kiwifruit improves bowel function in patients with irritable bowel syndrome with constipation. *Asia Pac J Clin Nutr.* 2010;19(4):451–457.

Chey SW, Chey WD, Jackson K, Eswaran S. Exploratory comparative effectiveness trial of green kiwifruit, psyllium, or prunes in US patients with chronic constipation. *Am J Gastroenterol.* 2021;116(6):1304–1312.

Chiba T, Kudara N, Sato M, et al. Colonic transit, bowel movements, stool form, and abdominal pain in irritable bowel syndrome by treatments with calcium polycarbophil. *Hepatogastroenterology.* 2005;52(65):1416–1420.

Lambeau KV, McRorie JW Jr. Fiber supplements and clinically proven health benefits: How to recognize and recommend an effective fiber therapy. *J Am Assoc Nurse Pract.* 2017;29(4):216–223.

McRorie JW Jr. Evidence-based approach to fiber supplements and clinically meaningful health benefits, part 2. *Nutr Today.* 2015;50(2):90–97.

Mounsey A, Raleigh M, Wilson A. Management of constipation in older adults. *Am Fam Physician.* 2015;92(6):500–504.

Mueller-Lissner SA, Wald A. Constipation in adults. *BMJ Clin Evid.* 2010;0413.

Musso CG. Magnesium metabolism in health and disease. *Int Urol Nephrol.* 2009;41(2):357–362.

Pare P, Bridges R, Champion MC, Ganguli SC, Gray JR, Irvine EJ, Plourde V, Poitras P, Turnbull GK, Moayyedi P, Flook N, Collins SM. Recommendations on chronic constipation (including constipation associated with irritable bowel syndrome) treatment. *Can J Gastroenterol.* 2007;21(Suppl B):3B–22B.

Rao SSC, Brenner DM. Efficacy and safety of over-the-counter therapies for chronic constipation: An updated systematic review. *Am J Gastroenterol.* 2021;116(6):1156–1181.

Soltanian N, Janghorbani M. Effect of flaxseed or psyllium vs. placebo on management of constipation, weight, glycemia, and lipids: A randomized trial in constipated patients with type 2 diabetes. *Clin Nutr ESPEN.* 2019;29:41–48.

Sun J, Bai H, Ma J, et al. Effects of flaxseed supplementation on functional constipation and quality of life in a Chinese population: A randomized trial. *Asia Pac J Clin Nutr.* 2020;29(1):61–67.

Chapter 11

Good MM, Solomon ER. Pelvic floor disorders. *Obstet Gynecol Clin North Am.* 2019;46(3):527–540.

Haylen BT, de Ridder D, Freeman RM, Swift SE, Berghmans B, Lee J, Monga A, Petri E, Rizk DE, Sand PK, Schaer GN. An International

Urogynecological Association (IUGA)/International Continence Society (ICS) joint report on the terminology for female pelvic floor dysfunction. *Neurourol Urodyn*. 2010;29:4–20.

Lacerda-Filho A, Lima MJR, Magalhães MF, Paiva RDA, Cunha-Melo JRD. Chronic constipation—the role of clinical assessment and colorectal physiologic tests to obtain an etiologic diagnosis. *Arquivos de Gastroenterologia*. 2008;45(1):50–57.

Lee HJ, Boo S-J, Jung KW, et al. Long-term efficacy of biofeedback therapy in patients with dyssynergic defecation: Results of a median 44 months follow-up. *Neurogastroenterol Motility*. 2015;27(6):787–795.

Patcharatrakul T, Rao SSC. Update on the pathophysiology and management of anorectal disorders. *Gut Liver*. 2018;12(4):375–384.

Rao SS, Go JT. Treating pelvic floor disorders of defecation: Management or cure? *Curr Gastroenterol Rep*. 2009 Aug;11(4):278–287.

Rao SS. Dyssynergic defecation and biofeedback therapy. *Gastroenterol Clin North Am*. 2008;37(3):569–586.

Skardoon GR, Khera AJ, Emmanuel AV, Burgell RE. Review article: Dyssynergic defaecation and biofeedback therapy in the pathophysiology and management of functional constipation. *Aliment Pharmacol Ther*. 2017;46:410–423.

Wallace SL, Miller LD, Mishra K. Pelvic floor physical therapy in the treatment of pelvic floor dysfunction in women. *Curr Opin Obstet Gynecol*. 2019;31(6):485–493.

Yeo CJ, Keller DS, Silviera M. Pelvic Floor Dysfunction. In: *Shackelfords Surgery of the Alimentary Tract*. Vol 2. 8th ed. Elsevier; 2019:1750–1760.

Chapter 12

Chiba T, Kudara N, Sato M, et al. Colonic transit, bowel movements, stool form, and abdominal pain in irritable bowel syndrome by treatments with calcium polycarbophil. *Hepatogastroenterology*. 2005;52(65):1416–1420.

Lambeau KV, McRorie JW Jr. Fiber supplements and clinically proven health benefits: How to recognize and recommend an effective fiber therapy. *J Am Assoc Nurse Pract*. 2017;29(4):216–223.

Manitius N. Fiber for Inflammatory Bowel Disease (patient education handout). Dietitians in Medical Nutrition Therapy, a dietetic practice group of the Academy of Nutrition and Dietetics. 2021.

Soltanian N, Janghorbani M. Effect of flaxseed or psyllium vs. placebo on management of constipation, weight, glycemia, and lipids: A randomized trial in constipated patients with type 2 diabetes. *Clin Nutr ESPEN*. 2019;29:41–48.

Sun J, Bai H, Ma J, et al. Effects of flaxseed supplementation on functional constipation and quality of life in a Chinese population: A randomized trial. *Asia Pac J Clin Nutr.* 2020;29(1):61–67.

Chapter 13

Kishida K, Martinez G, Iida T, Yamada T, Ferraris RP, Toyoda Y. d-Allulose is a substrate of glucose transporter type 5 (GLUT5) in the small intestine. *Food Chem.* 2019;277:604–608.

Lenhart A, Chey WD. A systematic review of the effects of polyols on gastrointestinal health and irritable bowel syndrome. *Adv Nutr.* 2017;8(4):587–596.

Monash University FODMAP Diet app. Version 3.0.8 (434). Monash University.

QOL Medical. Accessed December 5, 2021. https://www.sucraid.com/.

Acknowledgments

I am grateful to many people whose encouragement, support, input and wisdom helped me bring *REGULAR* to life. I owe a huge thank-you to my beloved agent, Carole Bidnick, whose gentle probing around "What are you working on?" lit my proverbial fire and got me to finish this project. I'm grateful to my editor, Dan Ambrosio, for finding *REGULAR* a happy home at Hachette Go, and for having believed in my potential as an author years ago, even before I was one! I'm thrilled we finally got to work together. Thanks to Ville Mehtonen of Mehtonen Medical Studios for rendering this book's illustrations so precisely and artistically, and for being such a flexible, talented and generous collaborator.

Thank you to my brilliant and cherished physician colleagues who generously reviewed chapters of this book to ensure medical accuracy: Eric Goldstein, MD, Yevgenia Pashinsky, MD, and Asher Kornbluth, MD, of New York Gastroenterology Associates (NYGA); and Jennifer Toh, MD, of New York Allergy and Asthma. Thanks also to Drs. Jamie Aisenberg, James George, Leon Kavaler and the physician partners and providers at NYGA for entrusting me with our practice's patients, many of whose stories are embedded within these pages. To my outstanding dietitian colleagues at NYGA, Suzie Finkel, Shira Hirshberg and Faith Aronowitz: thank you for joining me on the dream team of GI dietitians.

I am blessed to have the most patient husband and forgiving children. M&S: unfortunately, the reward for your patience is the potential social humiliation of having a mom who writes books about pooping. At least I didn't dedicate the book to you this time, though, right? I love you, Alex, for many reasons, including for not batting an eyelash when I talk about poop at the dinner table or at parties, and of course also for keeping our family fed, clothed and alive (me included) while I was writing.

Index

abdominal pain, 20, 40, 50, 137, 208, 209
ALCAT testing, 64
alcohol, GI symptoms and, 49, 65, 66, 113, 131, 182
allulose, 265
amylase, 25
anal fissures, 18
anal pain, 20
anal sphincter, 224
anaphylaxis, 167–168
anismus, 225
anorectal manometry, 213, 226–227, 233
anorectal muscle dysfunction, 211
antibiotics, 76–77, 111, 141
anti-CdtB antibodies test, 51
anticholinergics, 74
antidepressants, 46, 76, 170
antidiarrheals, 75, 141
antihistamines, for histamine intolerance, 176–177

anti-inflammatory diet patterns, 148–159
  exclusive enteral nutrition, 148–149
  Mediterranean diet, 156–159
  partial enteral nutrition, 149–153
  specific carbohydrate diet, 153–156
antispasmodics, 74
anti-transglutaminase antibody test, 118
anti-viculin antibodies test, 51
artificial food coloring, avoiding foods with, 181–182
atypical food allergies, 65
autoimmune diseases, GI, 115, 134, 140, 155

bacteria
  in gut, 24, 26 (*see also* gut microbiota)
  in stool, 4–5

banding, for hemorrhoids, 17
basophilia, 169
basophils, 167
behavioral therapy, for managing
    IBS-D, 77–80
beverages
  low-histamine, 185
  simple carbohydrate levels in
    various, 258, 262, 268
bidets, 16
Bifidobacterium sp., 70–71
bile, 5, 25, 98, 104
bile acid diarrhea (BAD), 26, 28,
    98–103, 104, 134
bile acid malabsorption (BAM), 25,
    98–103
bile acids, 25, 98–99
bile acid sequestrants, 101–102,
    103
bilirubin, 5
biofeedback therapy, for pelvic
    floor dysfunction, 228
biologics, 141
biphasic diet, SIBO and, 115
The Bloated Belly Whisperer
    (Freuman), 32, 56, 103
bloating, 107, 171, 209
blood in stool, 20, 136
blood tests
  to diagnose celiac disease, 118
  to diagnose histamine
    intolerance, 174–175
  to diagnose IBD, 139
  to diagnose IBS-C and slow
    transit constipation, 210
  to diagnose IBS-D, 49
body weight, fiber intake and, 197
bone density, corticosteroids and,
    159–160

bone density scan (DEXA), celiac
    disease and, 127
bowel, 11
  alarm symptoms, 20
bowel movement, 3
  frequency of, 7
  waking overnight to have, 20,
    38, 48, 87, 97, 101, 136
bowel obstructions, 19, 134
bowel patterns, questions about, 37
bowel regimen, 213, 230
brain-gut axis, 22–23
breakfast, sending motility message
    to colon and, 220
Breaking the Vicious Cycle
    (Gottschall), 153
breath testing, 64, 88–90, 108–110
Bristol Stool Chart, 7–10
  artist's reproduction of, 9

calprotectin, 137
Campylobacter, 50
capsule endoscopy, 138–139
carbohydrate-conscious eaters
  case study of constipation from
    fiber imbalance, 205–206
  sample balanced fiber diet for,
    203–204
carbohydrate intolerances, 55
  managing symptoms of,
    255–256
  masked by constipation, 94–96
  sugar-restricted diets for people
    with multiple, 276–278
carbohydrate malabsorption, 55,
    84, 86–87, 90–94. *See also*
    osmotic diarrhea
carcinoid tumors, 169
Case, Shelley, 125

low-lactose and lactose-free diet, 256–260

low-sucrose diet, 266–272

low-sugar alcohol/polyol diets, 272–276

lubricants, 216

magnesium, as laxative, 28, 201, 206, 209, 214, 230

magnetic resonance enterography (MRE), 139

malabsorption, 11
  bile acid, 25, 98–103
  carbohydrate, 55, 84, 86–88, 90–94

malnutrition, 147. *See also* nutritional deficiencies

maltase, 25, 82–83

maltose intolerance, osmotic diarrhea and, 82–84, 85

maltose malabsorption symptoms, 86–87

mannitol, 85, 273, 276

mast cell disorders, 169

mast cells, 167, 174

mast cell stabilizers, for histamine intolerance, 178

meal/portion size, GI symptoms and, 54–55, 146, 221

meat, histamine and, 180–181

mechanics of digestive transit. *See* digestive transit, mechanics of

medical approaches
  for histamine intolerance, 176–178
  for IBD, 139–142
  for IBS-C and slow transit constipation, 213–219

for osmotic diarrhea from carbohydrate malabsorption, 93–94

medical approaches to manage IBS-D, 74–77
  antibiotics, 76–77
  antidepressants, 76
  antidiarrheals, 75
  antispasmodics, 74

medications
  gluten-free diet and, 125
  sugar alcohol levels in various, 276

Mediterranean diet, 152, 155–159

menus, sample
  gentle fiber/GI gentle diet, 252–253
  low-histamine diet, 187–188
  Mediterranean diet, 156–157
  soluble fiber-rich or fiber-predominant diet, 246–247
  for specific carbohydrate diet, 154

metabolic rate, 13

metabolism, misconceptions about, 12–13

metabolome, 29–30

Methanobrevibacter smithii, 106

methanogenic SIBO/methane-predominant SIBO, 106

minerals, in stool, 5

mixed/eight-strain probiotics, 162–163

mixed-type IBS (IBS-M), 94

morning routine, to manage IBS-C and slow transit constipation, 220

mornings, digestive symptoms in, 39, 47–48